A SERIES OF ELEVEN LESSONS

IN

KARMA YOGA

(THE YOGI PHILOSOPHY OF THOUGHT-USE)

AND

THE YOGIN DOCTRINE OF WORK

By BHIKSHU

The kingdom of Thought is truly yours; you can select values, reject vanities, eliminate dross, live as the uncrowned and crowned Emperors have lived in the utmost independence, ordering for yourself Happiness, distributing the flowing surpluses thereof to all around you.

CHICAGO, U. S. A.

YOGI PUBLICATION SOCIETY

1928

INDIA AGENTS:

THE LATENT LIGHT CULTURE, TINNEVELLY. (S. INDIA.)

ISBN 0-911662-20-0

PRINTED IN THE UNITED STATES OF AMERICA

PUBLISHERS' NOTE

The lessons included in this book are written by an Asiatic for the English speaking peoples of the world, and suffer from the fact that the mother tongue of the writer is not English nor Sanskrit and that his metaphysic is oriental. Much of the teaching that is given here has been given out privately in the Yogaic schools of the select, though not in the practical form herein presented. The excuse for the book is the need of arrangement before doubting, enquiring minds prepared to question every argument and assertion; of facts and theories so that they fit in with the composite scheme presented by the Yogi philosophy.

The publishers take the liberty to call the attention of the reader to the great amount of information *condensed* in the space given to each lesson. Students have told us that they have found it necessary to read and study each lesson carefully in order to absorb the varied information contained within its pages. They have also stated that they have found it advisable to re-read the lessons several times allowing an interval between each reading, and that at each re-reading they would discover information that had escaped them previously during the study. This has been repeated to us so often that we feel justified in mentioning it that other readers might avail themselves of the same course and plan of study.

One other matter: The book is intended to be completed by the personal interest of the reader and his desire to know the teachings better, a desire that the Latent Light Culture is prepared to meet freely; we do not take leave of the reader in presenting the book to him, we desire better acquaintance as we are also seekers of the Light.

LATENT LIGHT CULTURE

Agents of the Yogi Publication Society in India.

Table of Contents

Thought the builder; The universe, of thought, of the dead that are living; Brief description of death and after; The need of interchange of intercourse with the plane of the dead.

Lesson IX

All worship began as the worship of the dead; The offer of *thilah*, good thoughts, and *akshatas* undying affection to the *manes*; The *tarpana*; The fire mystery; The use of incense; the modern fire worship suggested; The Lord's prayer and *Fateha*; The obligations to other lives in Nature; The Eucharist; The duty to the Universal Mind, *Brahma*.

Lesson X

The Karma Yogi that has got beyond selfishness; The modern problem; The substitute for Asceticism; Vicarious suffering; The East requires a different praxis; Schemes for the Western (*Vani*) social worker; His ideal to be the Sun; Sun worship; A *mantra*.

Lesson XI

The dullness in Karma Yogi's life; The power of cumulation; Dryness; The Air trial, without programme; Reversion; The task one of changing the center; The need for watchfulness.

PEACE TO ALL BEINGS

KARMA YOGA

LESSON I

It was said by Yogi Ramacharaka (p. 117 of the *Advanced Course in Yogi Philosophy and Oriental Occultism*) that "many western seekers after truth have complained that the philosophies of the East were not adapted to the needs and requirements of the westerner, as the conditions of life were different in the two different parts of the world". . . The trouble with these objecting western students is that they have considered the eastern teachings to be fit only for those who could spend their life in dreaming, meditation and in seclusion far away from the busy life. But this is a great mistake. Every true Yogi recognizes that even in the East a life of activity is right and proper for those who are thrown into it, and that to shirk its duties or run away is a violation of the great *Law Dharma* called also "God's Law." And to that end is herein pointed out the beauties and advantages of that important branch of Yogi philosophy and praxis known as "Karma Yoga."

The phrase "Karma" Yoga has passed through many vicissitudes in its meaning which has changed from time to time, and from creed to creed, till now it is treated as equivalent to what is known as the Doctrine of Non-attachment. In the East, in India especially, due to the peaceful occupation by the governing race, the depressing fact has come to prevail that so many Indians will do just what the actual requirements of their vocation demand and nothing else, unless the State makes it worth their while. To these, as also to the western peoples who on their part have to learn to appreciate more than ever the meaning of equanimity, to subdue their feverish haste with a little more evenness of the mind, the following lessons on the need of a new orientation towards the Doctrine of Work, KARMA YOGA, are issued.

The word "Karma" has been derived from the Sanskrit root "Kr" meaning "to effect" and it is interesting to trace the history of the word Karma. At about the time that the *Bhagavad Gita* was taught in its original form, there prevailed, even in that antique period, doubts as to what *was* Karma and what, not—and the Lord Krishna settled the doubts by suggesting that Karma in brief was the emanation (*Visarga*) that gave rise to the Ideas (*Bhava*) which taking shape or form came to be (*Bhoota*) (*Bhagavad Gita*, VIII-3). Later teachers and religionists commenting here-. on made it out that "Karma" referred to the acts enjoined by the Sacred Scriptures of *their* times and taught that "Karma Yoga" was the adoption of the religious life and praxis of Yoga as ordained thereby, against the perversion and exaggeration of which teaching still later thinkers said that "Karma Yoga" meant only submission to the duties and responsibilities of the normal life, which duties and responsibilities the Yogi was always to recognise; and the Yogi was not to feel enamoured of the life of the cloister or of the wanderer. In its most modern sense, the Karma Yogi is the Yogi who whether a *Gnani Yogi* or *Bhakti Yogi* or *Raja Yogi* or no Yogi at all, is still a Purposeful man or woman, having settled views, a *Grihee* (householder) practising Yoga while actively in with the world's turmoil; and it is in this sense that we shall take the phrase "Karma Yogi" and a scheme of life for such a "Karma Yogi" to be *Karma Yoga*.

Prince Siddharta who was Gautama the Buddha (Enlightened) said the very same thing as did Krishna; in the first twin verses of the *Dharma Pada*, he says, "All that we are is the result of what we have thought, it is founded on Thought, it is made up of our thoughts. If a man acts or speaks with an evil thought, pain follows him as the wheel follows the foot of the ox that draws the chariot." This is the world renowned *"Law of Karma,"* the law that is the fullest application of the Christian teaching that "as you sow you shall reap," the scientific axiom "that action and reaction are equal and opposite," pushed to its logical conclusions on the planes of thought that govern, regulate and underlie action. To the Buddhists this Law of Karma stands pragmatically for the God of the Theists and for much more; for, whereas in the Christian religion, as in Islam, God can override "Karma" by His Great Power of Mercy, in Buddhism and in Jainism Karma can in no sense be appeased; evil *must* be suffered by pain; good acts *are* rewarded by subsequent pleasures. There is no way out of the situation than to submit to Karma, and to make the best of it, realising thus the meaning and use of pain, says the Jaino-Buddhist view.

This law of Karma governs the horizon of view of the ethics of the Asiatic peoples, regulating the ethics with its very stern hand. The Jain owes his transcendental altruism, whereby he forbears from injury of every living creature and prays periodically for forgiveness from sins unconsciously committed, entirely to his basic Law of Karma. To the Jain, man is continually by his actions pouring forth a "Karma" that *colors* him and colors his vision, that goes into his being and in time spends itself, in the reaction of effect equal to the cause, as pain or pleasure. The Jain carries his altruism so far as to maintain a rest house for aged domestic animals where they may die peacefully; he carries it so far as not to burn lights in his house lest moths be attracted thereby and die therein; he avoids taking meals at night so that living creation of the minute nocturnal type may not be interfered with; nay he even discourages travel during the rainy season when animalculae spring up everywhere in the tropical lands. Both the Jain and Buddhist have built up a most elaborate code of ethics, of what to do and what not, all based on the Law of Karma, and they have also divided themselves communally into the two classes, the laity who *recognised* the Law of Karma, and the priesthood who *abided* by the Law, subjecting their Rules of Life to the Law.

The Hindus, however, retained their antique modes of life while recognising the Law of Karma. To them the law of Action and Reaction was paramount and conformance to the law necessitated the observance of a code of ethics which, however, they made very complex, and extremely elaborate. Mankind, said the Hindu, was to be found in four classes: (1) *Brahmins*, Priests, workers with God, or workers with the Law, (2) *Kshatriyas*, rulers, warriors, maintaining the Law, (3) *Vaisyas*, artisans and agriculturists abiding by the Law and (4) the *Panchamas*, the slaves or serfs outside the pale of the Law, who knew not the good Law, or would not abide by it, and thus

continued slaves. Each class had its own code of
conduct, its own rules of life; and so long as each
member observed these rules, he was free to continue to be a member of his class, with the re-
wards and punishments, rights and responsibilities thereof, and free to enjoy the "club" life of
his class in each commune. Any member of any
class may take up any occupation of any class
lesser than he in the social rank which was, of
course, governed by birth, but whether he would
be accepted as member of such lower class depended on the goodwill of the community whose
occupation he was taking up; certainly he could
not remain a member of his own community
thence-after. Nor could any one easily take up
the profession of a higher class *at all*; Hindus, it
has been observed, did not endeavour to admit
proselytes, because their religion depended much
less on creed in which they are latitudinarians
than upon the fixed customs of their "castes,"
the character of which customs, being derived from
birth, could not be transferred to strangers.

It cannot be forgotten that the orderly state of
the community suggested by the caste system of
the Hindus was governed by scriptures that recognised the rights and duties of men to each other,
of men to animals and plants, as well as to all
dumb living existence, of men to the mightier
Powers manifested or latent in Nature, in Fire,

Air, Water, Earth as well as in the Thoughts of Men. For generations, in various tongues, as the ancient people moved on, from Egypt, and Persia (Iran) to India and the Further East, they saw, and sang of how man should act towards the world around him, of how he should praise glory and appease power, of how he must put down evil and nourish the good; and they chanted it and taught it all in the *Gathas*, in the *Vedas*, in *Puranas* and in many other forms of poetry and prose. The text books of the Karma Yoga of the ancients were legion, but the teachings thereof are still living and we shall enquire into their rationale and use the best of what is available to us.

Look you, in very ancient times they did not call on any God at all! In the beginning, said they, was the Deed, (the Act)! There was no God necessary to stand intermediary between the Act and its effect (reward or punishment). Every Act had its effect or Reaction, equal and opposite; yes, equal and *opposite*. Herein is the evidence of all Scriptures which say in effect, "thus did they," "thus sang they," "thus thought they," "thus" as in these *Puranas*, relating of noble deeds and valiant conduct, "thus" as in these phantasies and songs of the *Gita* and *Gatha*, *Vedas* and (*Zend*) *chandas*; "thus" as in the heights of speculation of the *Upanishads* and *Brahmanas*. "Go *thou*, then, neophyte 'Karma Yogi' and *do like-wise*. Sing thou chants like unto the ancient chants, sing thou out the joy or pain in thyself, but let it be a *song;* work thou out deeds or *the* deed before you as the best of them, learned in the law, would do, as the ancients are said to have done; think thou out the thoughts of the *Upan-ishads*, of how thoughts themselves lose in the stillness of silence all their sting and return strengthened to solace the aching soul."

"The forging of earthly chains," says a Master, "is the occupation of the indifferent. It is folly to re-duplicate these by persistent regrets for the past, by present cowardice or by fear of the fu-ture. It is eternity that man mistakes for Past, Present and Future." You are what you did in the past, you here are Lord of the present, your future will be inseparable from yourself. Such is the teaching of the Hindu-Yogi Philosophy which combines both Freewill and Predestination in its excellent system of ethics and in its world scheme. *Predestined* are you by the weight of force of your own *Karma*, your past Acts (Thoughts, words, deed); *Freewill* have you such as you are, to Act; and you will be *as* you *Act now*. "As you sow you will reap" is truly an uni-versal axiom which the Christian takes to refer to this world of effects only, whereas the Hindu takes it to have force on the moral plane governing the physical, as well. *Act* Thou, therefore, when opportunity confronts you; responding to it, meeting it bravely, utilising it, actively. "*Do* what thou wilt," say the Masters, "Shalt be the whole of the Law," of Dharma of Karma—only he who *doeth* is the Karmi; he who *wills to do* and doeth is the Karma Yogi; the *Deed* is the *Karma*, his future, his Destiny the harvest of his Thoughts and Acts. Your Deed is the expression of your will, the will in you; say then to yourself "I will" and Act. So acting shalt thou not sin, says the Lord Krishna.

On no account hesitate. The Yogi teachers are very distinct on this point. Reflect, certainly, before the Act, but let not indecision foul the Reflection. If the authors of the French Revolution had been arguing it out, repeating, reflecting, doubting, hesitating about the consequences or about the Act, the expression of their High Principles, they would have become gray-haired without accomplishing anything. "The doubter perishes," says the Hindu Yogi, he rots, becomes good for nothing. Alas, doubt is the characteristic of the majority of persons, men whose actions cancel each other out. One goes on from day to day doing a little of this and a little of that, thinking a few kind and a few unkind thoughts but not thinking any thought at all out thoroughly. Nothing gets done indeed till nightfall and body and mind are changed, changed beyond recall. What meaning hath any of this change, asks a Yogi. The doubter is really an ignorant person, in many ways, for he doubts the efficacy of the un-erring Karmic Law, the Law of Righteousness (Dharma) on which all the universe is founded; he doubts *himself,* he doubts whether he who can think, who *has* to act, can act; he doubts the world around, he doubts the great Purpose of Nature, of Nature that thrills with Motion, with Activity, that buds out and expands, becomes great and greater (*Brahma*) continually, always. And what after all is Doubt but *Asradha,* want of Faith, weakness of the will, evidence that the man is puny, that his "I" is the "I" of a weakling, of a decrepit, of a coward, not of a God, not of a Lord of crea-tion born with the Right to Act, that man is.

In this then shall be the Ordinance (*Sastra*) for you Karma Yogi, in the dictum of "Do what thou wilt" which shalt be for thee the whole of the law, teaching you comprehensively what to do, what to avoid, this the *only* ordinance; "do what thou wilt, then do nothing else"; we shall repeat it con-stantly, without end, that you may be unified of will, that in all your act you may bring all the uni-verse that is of you, that in your act the whole of you and not the puny portion of you miscalled the "I" at the threshold, at the outer gate of consciousness, may act, and impress itself on the event that anyhow must be.

And it is an excellent thing no doubt to make up your mind definitely; it gives all your arguments a certain sharpness, a certain definiteness till a point is reached and in time reached automatically, habitually, at which they suddenly issue forth to produce a definite result; and herein look you it is a matter of comparative indifference whether your ideations are true or not, whether your ideas are exact representations of the thing; what is of the highest importance is that whatever you believe in, should be believed to be true; the Hindus speak, from very ancient times, specially about this; they distinguish between *Rita* what is accepted as true and hence is superior, more useful, more effective than Truth, *Satya;* God himself in the Hindu concept is the Truth that is greater than truth.

Says the *Gita,* each man shall have only the value, the Power that is equivalent to his *Sradha,* his Faith, that is to say, only that portion of man's mental makeup is to be taken into our calculations as effective as is the sum total of his settled convictions, of his will to power, *Sradha.* Says the *Taittiriya Upanishad;*—"Of the *Vijnanamaya* sheath of man that interpenetrates the mental sheath (*Manomaya Kosha*) *Sradha,* the Believing in order to know is the head; *Rita,* the judgment

as to whether anything is proper or righteous, is
the tolerant (*dakshina*) view; Truth is its saving
(*uttara*) aspect; application (Yoga) is its embodiment (*atma* or self); its remainder is greatness
(*Mahah*)."

Of course the ancient Sanskrit is difficult to
translate into modern Sanskrit and harder still to
translate into modern English, but what may be
stated is that man is considered as a composite of
an essence with five coats, of which the outermost
is experience (*Anna*), the next life (*Prana*), the
third mentality (*Manomaya*), interpenetrating all
of which is the Higher Man, the transcendent portion of man, of the thinker out-of-the-herd, called
Vijnana. Such a man believes a thing not because
it is true but because it has to be believed to be
true for the purpose of the Act-necessary; this is
his *Sradha;* the faith that moves mountains.
Such a faith should not go *against truth;* it may
transcend the literal truth, but truth is its saving
grace (*uttara paksha*); such a faith is founded on
the charity of righteousness; it is countenanced
just because, for the sake of righteousness, for the
sake of the Act, it has to be believed in; a concrete instance would be the faith of the soldier
that killing the enemy in war is not slaughter.
And such a faith does find application in every-
day life; it finds ecstasy (*yoga*) in fulfillment, says
the *Upanishad*. And how Great the power of the

faith is can be seen, it is so great that it leaves greatness as its tail, as its remainder. Yes, this is the first lesson of the real useful Karma Yoga.

"As each one Believes shall he know and Be"

LESSON II

In very ancient times when the Indians and Iranians (Persians) aboded together, they had the same word for *Fire* or rather the same concept, which they translated later, the Iranians into *fire* and the Indians to *righteousness,* the root of the word *Rta.* In Parsi literature *rita* became *athar* (fire) and the fire priest was *atharvan;* the *atharvan* corresponding to the *rithvik* or *Brahmin;* and to the *angiras; angiras* being "son of fire" (*agni*). Both in Persia and in India the sense that there is something beyond this herd life to be attained, the desire to reach out to that life, was in all beings; it was the fire in them, *athar* in *Persia, rita* in India, *Dharma* in later and Buddhist-Hindu parlance; *Sradha* in its complete translation in Vedic times. Any one who desired ardently (the term "ardent" is phonetically from the same origin as *rita, arta,* and *athar*) attained it, for that was the *Dharma,* the Law, the *Talmud* (Dharma's code). We find the word *sradha* to be of very ancient origin as a concept; it is the "creed" of the English, the faith to which he subscribes as to the flag he serves under, it is the "credo" of the Latin, the "cretin" of the Slavic, the faith to which according to the Hindu scriptures he shall devote himself every morn on rising up whether the Sun himself has risen or not. As says the Hindu text, having devoted yourself to the work before you for the day, having taken care to exclude vanities of no use whatsoever for the day, draw up your programme to which you shall devote yourself, devote yourself wholly as if it was your creed, as if it was your joy and your *necessity*, have not only any doubts hereabout at all.

There is further danger in this "Doubt" in that it is a division of the will. We would remind our students of the First Principles of the Hindu-Yogi Philosophy, as regards Man, namely that he is not a unity at all: (1) Every individual is a permanent organisation consisting of an indefinite number of living entities, each of which has Thought, Will and Feeling, graded in a "hierarchy" ranging from the most vital and essential to the least vital and least indispensable; (2) the most "vital" entities in the hierarchy are those which have the most powerful determining action on the vital processes. They are also those which are most essential to the organisation. (3) These vital entities may during life be called soul-particles and together they make up the *soul* or Personality. (4) This soul of the human individual besides being polypsychic is composed of an indefinite number of streams (or threads) of consciousness co-existing in each of us, which can be variously and in varying degrees associated and disassociated, each soul particle being regarded as a thread or stream of consciousness.

Yes, multiple personality is the rule and not the exception—all mankind are like unto as this. Says Frater P.: "They wish a dozen careers and the force which might have been sufficient to attain eminence in one is wasted on many. They are null, they drift, they are the flotsam in the ocean of life, all because of *Indecision*. It is this Indecision that becomes Fear, the Dweller on the Threshold so graphically described by Lord Lytton in his *Zanoni;* fear of the world, fear of the future, fear of oneself, fear the greatest enemy on the path of the Yogi. Says H. P. Blavatsky in the *Voice of the Silence:* "Beware of fear that spreadeth like the black and soundless wings of the midnight bat, between the moonlight of thy soul, and thy great goal that loometh in the distance far away." Fear, says a Brother, is the first of the pylons (gates) through which one passes, in the Egyptian system of Yogi discipline; and of course is the first and worst enemy in all schools of Thought culture. No one can become Immortal, without eradicating Fear, says the Hindu. Indeed to the Hindu no one can become a recluse or ascetic, none can be "saved" unless he has transcended Fear.

For this there is a very good reason. Fear like most other depressing notes, such as anger, sorrow, passion, envy, breaks down the unifying Personality—the soul-particles become divided into two camps hostile to each other. For there has been a suppression of the will, there has not been that judgment which residing in the single governing cell (soul-particle) can weld the whole to effect an Act. For look you, the deciding Power, both will and judgment prove on careful analysis and study, not to be distributed through a large number of entities in the soul-body but to reside in a single cell. The will and judgment are the result of autocratic and not democratic decisions. The theory underlying these facts has been carefully expounded for westerners by Freud in his Psychology of the Group-mind—and man is after all a group-mind himself. Without the king, without the will, there is anarchy, crime, and there is again the sin of omission. For "doing nothing" is not entirely a harmless thing in every case; to refuse to save life is murder, in all decent systems of ethics or of unwritten codes. In continuing to be subject to Indecision, man becomes a rat, dog, pig, brute, idiot or devil. He truly does "die," does undergo metempsychosis at once, in effect; he does not continue to be a Man and can scarcely hope to become God.

This is what the Lord Krishna repeatedly urges in the *Bhagavad Gita*. *Fight*, Arjuna, says he; find thy joy and pain, thy loss and gain, victory or defeat in the battle, and know that it is not joy or pain, loss or gain, victory or defeat that you experience but the *Battle*, the Battle of Life that is around, within and *irrespective* of you. The Battle of Life waits for nobody, men live, die, or are born, enjoy or delight irrespective of the fact that the scoffer, the decrepit, the coward, the degenerate has not joined in the fray. These may wait, as the drunkard waits for the lamp posts he cannot avoid hitting his head at, and hope that the lamp posts may pass on, but—is it Life, is it not rather the backwater, the lapwater of froth and foam, of dirt and foulness that is left behind for the coward to bathe under and be soiled by? Not alone that in the Indecision an opportunity has passed, but that an Act of God has not come to be. An Act (of God), a Radiance should have manifested, should have illumined the battle; for the act, of every individual, that should have been has not been, and the Indecisive person has thus sinned or erred doubly, he has not paid his dues to the world or to himself. And he has gained nothing truly, for the God in him will not act so fully again, the God in him has gone to sleep, leaving him a riven cloud, befogged and dry.

Not that doubts should not assail anyone; it is no crime at all to be weak. Even Arjuna had his Indecision, his doubts, and hence the *Gita*.

Westerners may read McSwiney's "Principles of Freedom" very carefully many times. "Because of our human weakness, our erring minds and sudden passions, the most confident of us may at times find himself in the mud. What then will uplift him if he has been a weaver in principle as well as in fact? He is helpless, disgraced, undone. Let him know in time that we do not set up fine principles in a fine conceit that we can easily live up to them but in the full consciousness that we cannot possibly live away from them. That is the bed-rock truth. When the man of finer faith by any slip comes to the earth he has to uplift him a staff that never fails, and to guide him a principle that strengthens him for another faith, to go forth, in a sense that Alexander never dreamt of, to conquer new worlds. It is the faith that is in him and the flag he serves that makes a man worthy, and the meanest way may be with the highest if he be true and give good service. Let us put by the broken reed and craft of little minds and give us for our saving hope the banner of angels and the loyalty of gods and men."

The teachings of Karma Yoga can indeed have no value if they do not strengthen the weakling; they are not merely solatial; they are *not* at all! *obiter dicta* of doctrine; they do not teach of any mediator or intercessor ready to help man when up against evil, nor of a Providence that fights man's fight within himself, without man's joining the affray or against the coward. Whatever the Act (of course the right Act under the circumstances has been decided on) it should be *done* without further indecision, is the blazen cry of the Karma Yogi. You may take it that God has, as Jesus Christ, atoned for the sins of mankind but of what use is that great teaching to you who are He of the Great Act. Mahomed Rasul Alla (the Peace of God be on him) spake of the great glory of God but at the same time said that no one shall bear the burden of another; none other can act *your* Act. Zoroaster, the Emperor of the Dravidian Parsis, (probably you question our description) said that life should be a continuous Act of putting down evil, a continuous Battle with evil. His God was ever fighting the Devil, *Angra Mainyus*. Good word, good deed, good thought was his slogan, and every *Act* was and is of course *good*.

It is delusion, says the Hindu-Yogi Philosophy, to suppose that doing nothing has no effect. As we have said already, to refuse to save life is murder; as the Hindus say, to refuse to spread good thoughts in the world is doing harm by permitting wrong thoughts to foul the mental plane. Says Evelyn Underhill: "A good deal of the pseudo mysticism that is industriously preached at the present time is crudely quietistic. It speaks of the necessity of "going into the silence" and even gives lessons in subconscious meditation—a state of vacant placidity is attained in which he rests remaining in a distracted idleness and misspending the time in expectation of extraordinary visits, believes he is united with his Principle." The quietists, says Underhill, by a perversion and violation of Christian teachings produce deliberately a half hypnotic state of passivity. They remain from every interior and exterior act. Such a repose is treason to God; quietism blinds a man plunging him into that ignorance which is not superior but inferior to all knowledge; such a man remains in himself, useless and inert; a repose that is simply laziness—a forgetfulness of God, of one's neighbour, of one's self. About the same words may apply to the ascetic. The ascetic thinks that by reducing himself to the condition of a vegetable he is advanced on the path of evolution. Advance is in the direction of more continuous and untiring energy.

The object of those who counsel non-action, which is very much to the fore in the modern pseudo *sanyasins* and *bairagis* of India, is to prevent any inward cause arising so that when the old causes have died out there is nothing left. In order to escape the effects of action, of the Law of Karma, namely continued existence (birth, death and rebirth), they propose simply not to act or to come as near to that Ideal as possible. The ascetic life is advocated not only because it approximates a state of inaction and so tends directly to obliterate *Karma* (Law) but also because withdrawal from the world is a kind of insurance against being entangled in worldly desires which lead man astray from his true goal, Emancipation, to quote the words of an American. But this is quite unphilosophical, for every effect as soon as it occurs—whether man act or not—becomes a new cause and is always equal to its cause. Truly we may talk of renouncing the world but the world has to renounce us for inaction to be complete. If you do not act, you drift.

"Do what thou wilt," then, is the categorical imperative of the Hindu-Yogi Philosophy. How much better is this than the categorical imperative of Kant, which shouts "Do your duty" without being able to tell us what that duty is. Moralists had tried for ages to formulate a moral law which should be foolproof but had only succeeded in compiling systems of putrid morality. So it struck Kant, says a western writer, as a bright idea, to coin *his* categorical imperative "Do thine duty," a law which need not work at all; for there was no criterion of duty defined at all. The philosophy of Kant herein is nothing but the philosophy, if any, of that cant that has been the

bane of religious creeds since the beginning of
the world. All along have men in their jealousy
and vindictiveness made out codes, legislated for
other men, have framed elaborate manuals of
what to do and what not to do, assigned duties to
individuals and congregations by birth, calling
them natural duties, created castes, confusions,
rituals and what not so that the other man shall
remain a slave. They continue to suggest the
advisability of doing one's duty, of being true to
oneself, of not avoiding the work which nature
has ordained for them, from birth (!), but as to
how to decide between the comparative claims of
two conflicting duties is not taught at all in the
philosophy of religious cant.

Nor think that there are many duties assigned
to you either by birth or by convention. The
idea of "duty" does not exist in the Hindu religion at all in spite of vehement attempts made
to assert that stitching is the natural duty of a man
born of tailor parents, or shaving the natural
duty of a barber's son. There are those, of
course they are not barbers nor tailors but high
caste, exclusive Brahmins, who assert that the
tailor and barber will attain salvation only by
stitching and shaving. Yes, these slaves shall
serve, say they the lords, of creation, of caste; and
to that end they say that a cobbler shall worship
God only by his cobbling without any worship at

all, and a barber shall shave and not worship God
which worship of God is the privilege of Brahmins who alone have to be employed for a re-
muneration by the tailor and the cobbler and the
butcher and the barber, to worship God. No *duty*
at all exists anywhere on anyone's part, no obligation, no slavery in this world the kingdom of God.
Each one is *free* to live as he wilt, to do as he wilt,
joyously and luxuriously, and there is nothing in
the way of Freedom at all. You may be a tailor
by birth; no need is there for you to stitch at all;
certainly you have the heredity that you can
stitch very much better, you can make of stitching
an art, find your joy in stitching easier than most
others; but compulsion there is none on you to be
a tailor. You may become a priest and may do
very well, as a priest, better than most priests
born.

This imaginary restriction in the concept of
"duty" or "duties," has been called *"Karma
Bandha,"* the obsession that man is bound or con-
strained to act in a particular manner either by the
Ten Commandments or the Buddhist *Pancha
Shila,* or by the voluminous Hindu Scriptures, or
by the *Koran.* They call this *"Gharam"* in Islam,
considering it a thing from which one is unable
to free himself. The first and greatest of all
privileges is to have recognised the ordinance
"Do what thou wilt" as not at all in any way op-

posite to the Karmic Law "Action and Reaction
are equal and opposite"; thus does one become
free and independent, thus does one destroy all
fear whether of convention, of custom, of creeds,
of other men or of death itself. Says the
Upanishad: "it is not for the wife's sake but for
one's own sake that the wife is dear; it is not for
the children's sake but for one's sake that children
are dear to one, nor money is dear to one for
money's sake but for his own sake is money dear."
Duty *really* has no meaning at all to the average
citizen or man of the world who is prepared to
transcend it, to transcend his concepts of duty
where himself is concerned; duty in such cases
becomes a burden and where not borne, a bondage.

"Do what thou wilt shalt be the whole of the
Law" is the mantra of this lesson of *Karma Yoga*.
There is no law beyond "Do what thou wilt"—
Ishta Poorti—the ordinance is called in the *Vedas*.
The individual will such as it feels to be, has al-
ways the last word, the casting vote. Read verse
XVIII, 63 of the *Bhagavad Gita* which, as says
F. T. Brookes in his "Gospel of the Gita," should
be in very large print. Pray do not pass it by.
Yes, the Adept does what he wills, and allows
nothing to interfere with it. This was the or-
dinance long ago in *Ecclesiates* II, 7 to 10: "Go
thy way, eat thy bread with joy, and drink thy wine
with a merry heart. Let thy garments be always

bright and let thine head lack no ointment. Live joyously all thy days of vanity." Thus too does the Qoran say; it repeatedly asserts that its omnipotent Lord-God does not compel men to adopt one way or another; it leaves it to the choice of the individual. And Freewill has been the building stone of Buddhism (Wisdom's Religion), freedom to act, restrained only by oneself that self being the embodies, enshaped past-Acts. Act thou, therefore, for he only can act who has a perfect Self.

"DO WHAT THOU WILT SHALT BE THE WHOLE OF THE LAW"

LESSON III

The Hindu-Yogi Philosophy is nothing if it does not answer all the canons of fair criticism. This has been assured by the method of instruction called the *Samwada* or the dialogue, wherein the student can raise all kinds of objection before he submit to the utter obedience necessary in the earlier stages of Yoga. The "dialogue" it may be mentioned by the way, is the most ancient form of religious instruction to be found as in the Gilgamesh Epic of the Babylonians, in the Teutonic myths, in the chronicles of Zoroaster, as well as in the *Vedas*. And the dialogue is the result of the querying habit of man, a query that is naught but the crown of all gifts that has come down to man. This more or less developed power of gathering one's activities together, and unifying them in a conscious self that can look at itself in a mirror and see itself objectively, *is* given to *everyone*. This is the vivid, controlling attention-shifting selfconsciousness, the psychical side of cerebral integration, the tribunal before which the promptings of the primary conscious and repressed unconscious must come up for judgment.

It is quite right therefore for everyone to ask himself "What is this Karma or Act?" Where does it begin? Where does it end? Action and Reaction, you say, are equal and opposite; where then can action be avoided or rather can any act be done which does not provoke reaction? What are the factors of the act? Is there no difference between the consciously performed and the unconsciously performed Act or omission? If so, what? Is there not such a thing as the agent or instrument, the vehicle or the cause of the Act, itself the cause of the Actor? And who pray is the Actor? Is man the actor? If, as they say, the reaction is equal and opposite to the action, who is the enjoyer of the action? Does man live long enough to enjoy the reaction of all his acts? Yes, these and other questions, a very long chain of them are and have from time immemorial been asked by querying minds as to the "Act," and the Scriptures of all nations are full of answers, complete or incomplete, thereto.

A complete answer is to be found in the dialogue, *Bhagavad Gita.* For the purposes of these lessons only the acts of the conscious person are taken for analysis and the Gita says that every act is prompted by knowledge, *Jnana,* made up of the thing known, *Jneyam,* and the knower, *Parijnata.* And the Act may be said to include the instrument *Karana,* the Act, Karma and the actor *Karta.*

And going further, the Gita says that in the utmost analysis, for the fulfillment of any act, five factors are required—so say the most ancient thinkers too. These five are: (1) The sphere governed by or governing the Act, the limit of pervasion of the act and *ipso facto*, of its consequences, the *Adhishtanta* (2) The enjoyer of the act, *Akarta*, he who is affected by the utmost consequences of the Act, *Bhokta*, quite irrespectively of the Act or Actor (3) Various kinds of *modes* of the Act, the ways in which the Act takes effect, is performed, or exhibits itself, *cheshta* (4) Various kinds of the instruments or agents of the Act, the intermediaries or restrictions between the Actor and the Act, *Karana* they are called, and (5) *Daiva*, God, if you please, the unseen factor, the marginal error, the uncounted host, the catalyst or decatalyst, time, etc.—in so many forms does it appear.

For every Act, continues the *Gita*, whether it is performed by the body, by the tongue (as speech or utterance) by the mind (as thought), these remain *five* factors, the five Actors. The sages commenting on this text tell us that the limit of pervasion of the Act, its sphere, is the body itself, the body alone, and by the body is meant the entire "kingdom" subject to each individual, his passions, desires, hopes, longings, possessions, etc., all that he identifies himself with.

This is his sphere of action, rather the sphere of the Reaction that follows the Act inevitably. This is quite in accord with the discoveries of modern Relativity which tell us that force is a mathematical fiction, that nothing one can do can affect really any other but himself, that no two particles of matter ever come into contact, that when they get too close to each other they both move off. The Actor is not at all an Integrity but a multiplicity; this is the fundamental doctrine of the Yogi Philosophy. From time out of mind they have been inculcating this precept that the Ego is not the "I," that the "I" is but a puny figment of the waking memory, quite powerless to effect the tremendous result *called* the body and *known* as the universe. They have uttered it in the *Vedas*, heard it from the *Puranas* and learnt it from the *Gita*. How foolish then those men of incomplete insight who not caring to think deeply or at all, state that oneself alone is the actor.

Let me quote the definition of the consciousness of the self given by James in his Psychology text book: "The consciousness of self involves a stream of thought each part of which as "I" can remember those that went before and know the things that they knew, and (2) could emphasise and care permanently for certain ones among these as "me" and appropriate to these the rest. The nucleus of the "me" is always the bodily existence felt to be present at the time. Whatever remembered past feelings resemble this present feeling are deemed to belong to the same "me" with it. Whatever other things are perceived to be associated with this feeling are deemed to be part of the "me's" experience and of them certain ones which fluctuate more or less are reckoned to be themselves constituent of the "me" in a larger sense—such are the clothes, material possessions, the friends, honors, esteem which the person receives or may receive. This "me" is of course an empirical aggregate of things objectively known. The "I" which knows them cannot itself be an aggregate neither for psychological purposes need it be considered to be an unchanging metaphysical entity like the spirit or a principle like the Ego viewed as out of time. It is a thought at every moment different from that of the last moment but appropriative of the latter together with all that the latter called its own."

All the experiential facts find room in the above description of the "I" unencumbered with any hypothesis other than passing states of mind. It shows that the "I" is *not* an unity nor an integrity but a *multiplicity*, and a multiplicity it is, incalculable, both of the human form, a body built up of billions of living entities, an impermanent aggregation of living cells, and of the human soul itself, composite of quintillions of souls each and

all non-finite compounds of fragments of anterior
lives, a congeries diseased, teeming with many
purposes and places and yet in whom there is no
power to persist.

How are actions, Karma, caused, then? Says
the Hindu Yogi: "Action (*Karma*) is a constant
function in the universe—the lives in nature,
man's or world's nature always *effect* Karma, as in
ideomotor action called by us *avashah karma*, irrespective of an attention or attentive being, in the
Act caused." In the language of Einstein and
the Relativists, events are continually happening;
matter is a succession of events; the succession of
events, rather, was called matter in so far as matter was a logical construction that could be made
from a series of events, grouped together in virtue of their semblance and continuity. Not only
that, according to Bertrand Russel (*A. B. C. of
Relativity*, p. 122): "Every bit of matter, little
or small, is at the top of its own hill in the space-
time continuum; the hill is what we know about;
the bit of matter is assumed for convenience."
Again says he on p. 222 thereof: "It is true that
there are still electrons and protons that persist
but these are to be conceived as strings of connected
events like the notes of a song."

The world before us is then a world not of
things in motion but a world of *events*, wherefrom
we judge whether what comes before our vision

is a *Behaviour* (*Guna*) or whether it is only a representation to ourselves of our own Thought (*Karma*). And first of all we have to remember that every Act, every Thought is symbolic and not real. "When we say, 'we see a table,' we use a highly abbreviated form of expression," says Russell, p. 214 of the book above quoted, "concealing complicated and difficult inferences the validity of which will be open to question," (in a world of relativity because no two points of view are the same). As says Max Nordau: "In every act of consciousness man perceives a symbol of the object and never object itself." First of all in the subject, i. e. in the field of perception of the subject, the *Adhistana*, the whole universe is mirrored and digested, by the subject, who is hence called *Akarta*, a *Gita* term for enjoyer. In this perception which is a vibration, motion or force, and which after all is not distinguishable from matter, there is an effect, *Cheshta*, on the perceiver; and the effect is both simple, and compound, direct, and indirect, i. e. *via* an instrument or agent, a *Karana*. In fact all the forces in the universe known and unknown (destiny or *Daiva*) are, in every act of perception, acting on the subject.

So too in every Act (*Karma*). All the forces in the subject together with all the forces in the universe are acting on every Instant (event)! Every event is generated not out of some proceeding event (Actor or Cause), but out of a *whole situation* or complex of events, no *one* of which could be regarded as the cause of any event, says "Relativity"; this being a translation into modern English of the teaching in the *Bhagavad Gita* (XVIII, 16). It would be idle to argue herefrom a sole Actor, an unity; and it would be more correct to argue that it was a Multiplicity that was the Actor in every Act. As a great Brother says, "the cry of I am I is most especially of that which, above all, is not the 'I'."

This is specifically seen in the old adage, "Nature will out," no hetero-suggestion is ever successful says the physician Coue, "if it is opposed to the conscious tastes and desires of the subject"; nature is oftentimes found to constrain a man to act; ideas that occupy obsessingly the threshold of consciousness are bound to issue in action, the self playing consciously no part in such Acts; this is a truism made in group psychology. The will of the many, *in* man has no consideration for any but its own purpose; this has to be understood by the Karma Yogi. For while man is working day and night at some trival detail of his affairs, a giant force, the "Purpose of the many in him," Destiny you may call it, the nature of space-time in his neighbourhood as the Relativists term it, may be advancing *pede claudo* to overtake him.

You may say that this the Reaction of the Action inaugurated by man himself at some time previous; nay, it is not that alone; what reacts so far as there is reaction is only that conscious act of man's surface consciousness that may have acted, and we can see that there is no proportion therein. The reaction though equal and opposite to the Action is still too trifling a part of the future; as Destiny, *Daiva* it is only *one* of the factors of the Act in the future. The freewill of man, such as it is, remains always unimpaired.

The moral that the Jains drew from all this teaching was that it was well to avoid sinful act, for after "a man has done manifold actions that injured many lives, his pleasure-seeking relations took up all his wealth while the doer suffered in Hell for his sins." The people of the Vedic times drew the moral that the past was not to be regretted but to be recognised by the neophyte Karma Yogi as the work of *Kama*, heedless thought, and of *Manyu*, anger, by the mantra *"Kamo Akarshid Manyur Akarshid"* (*Kama* caused it; *Manyu* caused it). Anyway the past was not to be regretted at all.

It can therefore be seen that the Law of the equality of Action and reaction on the mental plane, has not such value to the Karma Yogi, he recognises that every Act is the act or function of the Many; that a Unity can never be the sole actor; that every action is not caused but truly effect. The Karma Yogi has to recognise that things cannot have happened otherwise than as they have; this is the teaching of the word "*Tatha*" the submission to *kismet* that characterised Prince Sidharta the Buddha and many others after Him. Further he is to recognise that this Karmic ledger of each one is a peculiar record the balance of which is struck only after death; he does not know at any date what is owed him nor to whom all he owes debts; it is all a mess—but so it is. It leaves him only one conclusion, that nothing can excuse his inaction in any event, that nothing can exonerate him, that *his* Free-will that is the Free-will of the many in him has always power to prevail and overpower, and that this power is exercisable by himself, i. e. by the King in him. The will and judgment are always the result of autocratic and never of democratic decisions, is a fact recognised in group psychology, and this constitutes the base of man's Free-will. It is a unification of many wills rather than a single will full cell in man.

Such ideas as that the Law of Karma is a blind Law, a stern justice that takes no note of men's motives, or of God's mercy, have to be given up as worthless teaching unfit for and inapplicable to the Karma Yogi of all men. Behind all the apparent suffering and pain and malice of the world the Karma Yogi especially if he be the sufferer sees transcendent beauty, thrilling energy, enduring love, and the utter radiance that enchants. And, most especially the Karma Yogi *cannot* be a Fatalist.

For purposes of this lesson it is enough to recognise that though thou doest as thou wilt, what is done is not done by thee but by many milliards of cells that are of thy make-up. Remember that every act is to be of many milliard cells not of that fiction called the I or Ego.

The Mantra shall be herein, as follows:—

"I shall act, yet not I, but the many that live in, that are of Me, for them shall I act so that they may find their longing and fulfilment. I shall DO IT that they may live their life which elsewise they could not."

LESSON IV

What finally in the utmost analysis is the Act or Karma? The *Gita* has a peculiar answer. Karma, says the Gita, is the emanation (*Visarga*) that is the generator (*udbhava kara*) of Images (*Bhava*) which become Beings (*Bhootas*). It would be insufficient to translate Karma by the word "Action"; we can see that the word is in the ultimate meaningless, for being the product of many actors, "action" can only be a "result" or an "event." Traced to the "individual" behind the Act we recognise the "motive" of the Act, the thought behind the Act, the thoughts which make up the Act, the thought, which, the Gita in its excellent analysis, calls an "emanation that is the generator of images." That is what Flammarion also tells us, in his great work on "Death and After" in three volumes. We would refer our readers to that book for the scientific proof of the theory that Thought is the generator of Images.

In the Yogi Philosophy, Thought is an emanation of the Mind (*Brahma*), mind being used in the sense of an universal principle which creates and sustains the world of sensations and through which alone the world can be interpreted. Mind as the power of sentience is no wise synonymous with brain, disposition, instinct, intellect, intelligence, reason, sense, soul, spirit, thought or understanding. Mind is conscious cognition; it itself is neither one of the vehicles nor a set faculty of mental consciousness but is a movable factor between the "Ego" and Ego here is taken as the threshold of the Act (of consciousness) each or any one of the Ego's vehicles. Mind is only coincident with the mental nature in an ideal situation. Mind is Being when and where Being is attentive and may be focused so low as in an infant's moron prejudices. That is how westerners have defined the Mind; but in the Hindu Yogi Philosophy, Mind is only one of the aspects or factors of *Manas*, the other being *Budhi*, Reason or the power of Judgment, both Insight and Intuition; *Chitta*, the thought-emanating center, *Antahkarana* the thought-absorbing faculty.

We are here concerned with the *Manas*, in its aspects of reception, selection and emanation of Thoughts. We have many facts to learn yet about the Mind beyond the western analysis of the Mind which divides the Mind into the Subjective Mind (subconscious) and the Objective Mind. We have to be very careful not to confound these two minds with the Manas of Hindu phraseology. They would rather correspond, the subjective with *Prana* and the objective with *Manah* (one of the four factors of *Manas*). In the province of *Karma Yoga*, our chief factor is the Power of

Thought, of conscious Thought; we have naught to do with unconscious cerebration nor with ideo-motor action *Avasah Karma*, for it is obvious that unconscious cerebration cannot form the subject of Yoga or be used at all. All the same we have to know that Thought is a *constant* function *irrespective* of the Ego. The *Bhagavad Gita* says that not for an instant can anyone remain without emanating Thought, consciously or unconsciously. Like respiration, or oxidation, thought is a constant process but unlike the former, irrespective of the subject. For ideas are essentially motor and if one occupies the field of consciousness to the exclusion of incompatibles it is bound to issue in action——the self does not play consciously any part in such acts——is the dictum of modern western psychology, too.

Indeed man is continually peopling space, the thought-world, with emanated thoughts, consciously and unconsciously. And by man we do not mean a puny Being whose only consciousness is a little flicker of waking consciousness itself comprising at any moment but an insignificant fraction of his total memory, but a Being with a consciousness extending and working over the whole range of his personality whether instinctively or deliberately. That Being does not like the former go out of existence every time man goes to sleep but simply turns his attention to vital processes founded at a time of life when he could not speak and before words or other symbols could be used to bring these processes under the purview of the ordinary waking memory. This is the real man, a Being endowed with a stupendous memory and activity and an almost unlimited command over vital processes, and even over physical processes, a man such as only rare illumined geniuses are ever aware of Being but which we all are, though we know it not.

Of this Great (*Brahma*) Being, Thought is a constant function as has already been said; thoughts are being constantly emanated irrespective of the "Self" or Ego. Each moment, groups of thoughts are being formed made up of "likes," *Sadrisa*, from out of thoughts already in space and those just being emanated. And these thoughts cannot be killed nor restrained at all even by the cleverest man; following the laws of group psychology, provisional beings (*Bhootas*) are being constantly formed out of the heterogeneous elements (thoughts) which for a moment become combined exactly as the cells which constitute a living body form by their re-union a new Being which displays characteristics very different from those possessed by each of the cells singly. That is why there arises difficulty in many practices of concentration. Half-knowledge, such as of many teachers suggests hetero-suggestive bases, which do not at all lead to success, they being opposed not only to the conscious tastes and desires of the subject but also because the Thought-Being created by ideomotor action has no consideration for any but its own purpose. The *Bhagavad Gita* explains this out fully in verses XVIII, 59 and 60, and also in verse III, 33.

Yes, all thoughts whether created from or passing into the depths of being go to the make-up of one's own character, one's self. And in the finale, it is the character that governs the function of Thought. A fundamental teaching of the Eastern Hindu-Yogi Philosophy as it is of the philosophy of the West, is that every conscious thought passes down to the lower stratum and then and there becomes an element of our Being partaking of our conscious energy and playing its part in determining our mental and bodily states. If it is a helpful thought, all the better. Such is how Coue and his school define the Power of Thought. According to Flammarion, "Every thought considered as an emanation of the thinker, a thread spun out by the soul (silkworm) is a *Guna* (Behaviour) and acts with more or less intensity virtually as an agent called material acts, as a projectile or stone and may project itself afar. If a man thinks of murder he emits into the atmosphere (of thought) a murder-element, that remains and returns to him." Imagine thought as it exists in man raised out of him and as an active and energetic Being endowed with an inner life of its own and you have but a feeble illustration of that which fills a whole region, a whole universe beyond Time.

How near we are to this grand Truth, that we are actually denizens of a universe of Thought-forms, that we are all each complex thought-forms compounded entirely of *Thought*, we have scarcely recognised, even amongst those of us that have been devoting attention to practices of meditation and Yoga. It has been the experience of many when meditating that they have been interfered with by particular kinds of Thought, apparently coming from nowhere. And against this interference there has, alas, been wasted a good deal of pious gassing by most *Acharyas*. They have found it easier to say "Be good and you will be happy"; they have continued to make many generalisations, to tell you that the mind is the bugbear of all philosophers, that every time it wanders it should be brought back by force (?) and reapplied to the object,—generally the object is Miss Kundalini with the tail in her mouth, to modern Hindu practitioners. They continue to analyse *Nirvana*, *Moksha*, *Dhyana*, and to explore Hindu metaphysics utterly. The poor practitioner continues to have pious platitudes trumpeted forth to him, continues to be fobbed off with inane remarks on virtue and Raja Yoga, Gnana Yoga, and such other *Rogas* (diseases) in his hour of need.

Be it well understood of you that it is not necessary nor right to shut off natural activity of any kind, (*Sahaja*). Thoughts (*Karma*) do as one sits to meditation come easily on before the threshold of consciousness, often times they are mean, clouded, inchoate, harmful; for in life there is much meanness (*dosha*); man is often called on to acknowledge some degrading standard or fight for the very recognition of manhood. And what is the remedy? How shall we get rid of these thoughts? The answer of the *Bhagavad Gita* is that you should *not effort* to take the trouble even of attempting to reject, much less to accept any of these thoughts; presently the thought atmosphere will clear, the smoke will disappear for the flame to burn brighter. Yes, if a man gets into a serious worry, it is doubtless well to face it and see what it means and to get expert advice such as the Latent Light Culture literature can give gladly, if the trouble does not smooth out. But in ordinary life it is probably better to leave the roots of the unconscious to look after themselves; it is better to try to grow some flowers or fruit including health of body and mind. When difficulties apparently insurmountable confront thee, all that thou has to do is not to fight it out without knowing what you fight against, but to wait and see, to calmly observe what it is. Perchance it may pass off; certainly it will clear, it will begin to work itself out and become less powerful.

A Russian confrere in translating the term *Parjanya* (the Rain God of the Occidental-Oriental) says that all that is seething in war, in the "struggle for existence," of passion, pain and the joy of victory is not only perceptible in its effects as revealed to the physical senses; it may be seen as an atmospheric process in the spirit world, a sort of thunderstorm. For each thought has a form, is a sort of cloud or mist and makes up in its electrical and magnetic potency a perfect analogue to a rain cloud. The simile is further expanded by Fournier D'Albe in his "New Lights on Immortality": "On the earth nearly a hundred-thousand persons die every day, the great majority of them being unconscious purposeless monads. The atmosphere is full of them. They remain for some time in the atmosphere and form a cosmic environment of diffused consciousness which mingles with the subconscious at time and manifests in mediumistic and spiritistic phenomena." These "monads" are of course the multiplicities of thoughts that were not expended with the body that had been shed, and they are only aggregations not certainly with any power of persisting as such but mere aggregations of thought-forms. Our point is here that the universe is peopled by these thought-forms and that it is quite possible for some of these thought-forms to appear before our consciousness as we sit to meditation or sit to think —all that you have to do is to wait, wait till they pass on.

As you can see for yourself, ideas are in the air around us; it is ideas that we see spread before us; spread before our consciousness, ideas that govern and move all things; guns, bayonets, men of war, aeroplanes are but outward symbols. These ideas are neither to be bayonetted or battoned down; they are not to be shot down either. You cannot of course disperse or kill ideas in this way— they thrive and sprout, aye, even, under the spilling of blood, *especially* under the spilling of blood. We have to deal with these Ideas or Thoughts in quite other ways. We have to recognise ourselves as not yet fully competent to deal single-handed, I mean with a superficial attention, with these ideas pouring on us. And different modes of treatment are prescribed for different forms of thoughts; it is impossible to frame a general law for dealing with *all* wrong thoughts, and attempts such as that of the categorical imperative of Kant or the "congenital duty" of the eastern pseudo-Yogi can only end in failure to grasp the principles of Karma Yoga.

As says Coue, "A form of particular suggestion (*Nirdesa*, the *Bhagavad Gita* calls it) is the *quiet* repetition of a single word. If your mind is worried and confused whether by the thoughts that had been oppressing you till you sat to meditation, or that had been pouring on you preventing your practice of mental-gymnastics for that day, *sit down,* close your eyes, relax yourselves, and murmur slowly and reflectively the single word (AUMN or) *calm*; say it reverently, drawing it out to its full length and pausing a bit after each repetition." And curiously Coue adds this method has been found most applicable to the attainment of *moral* qualities! It shows how powerful are some simple means and how independent of the ends actually attained. Each man may use *his* word, AUMN, Amen, Allah, as he likes—all that is necessary is to follow the direction given and to use the *Mantra,* we suggest the

A U M N

You may wonder how such a simple word can produce a development of the moral qualities! The reason is given by Freud, the psychologist who has specially analysed for us the workings of the Group Mind. "A group," he says, "is subject to the truly magical power of "names" or words; words can provoke the most formidable tempests in the group-mind and are also capable of stilling them!" And again, he says "Reason and argument are incapable of combating certain words or formulae. These words are uttered in solemnity in the presence of groups and as soon as they have been pronounced all heads are bowed with respect." Note this faculty of the group-mind carefully; realize herewithal that man's mind is after all a group-mind, that it is a collection of thoughts (many milliards of them), that it is a collection of thoughts (many milliards of them), that it is a collocation of these thoughts, and you will find reason enough to apply by analogy all the postulates of Group Psychology to the individual Human mentation.

Thus you see the AUMN in the auto-suggestion of *Karma-Yoga* to still all worries. But in the use of the AUMN do not seek for results, continues the *Gita*; do not expect any particular effect to follow on the utterance. To do so would first of all be to distract the attention and lessen the efficacy of the AUMN and secondly it would be a diversion *away* from the AUMN. Do the work of pronunciation or utterance of the AUMN and do nothing else. Avoid extensions of the thought suggested, if any, by AUMN by the very pronunciation itself; centralise entirely on the AUMN. Thus use *every mantra*, use it as an auto-suggestion, affirming it to yourself by repetition and not by forcing it on your subconscious. Let the AUMN in time form part of your Being replacing the thoughts of worry that had occurred, that may occur, unless superseded by the utterance of the AUMN. This was the word (sound) that was, that has to be, has to prevail and be uttered; in the beginning, it was the word that was with God, i. e. with what is beyond behind phenomena (such is the sense of "God" taken here), the word that is God (as far as our pragmatic experience goes), stilling all worries, solacing all griefs, as "God" the "God" of the cults can and does (still) solace.

LESSON V

Students must doubtless have studied and understood the significance and power of Thought, and that they may do it thoroughly is our object in this lesson. In dealing with conscious thought that is with thought arising from, or coincidentally with *Perception* or contact (*sparsa*), we have to remember the sevenfold nature of any Perception, e. g. the vision of a table. There is primarily the vision of the table with the sense of sight; secondly seeing it still with the eyes closed by retinal impression; thirdly the image of it conserved in the brain; fourthly it can be recalled by the memory; fifthly it can be seen in a dream; sixthly, or as an aggregate of its atoms or components, and seventhly as disintegrate. There are thus seven ways in which a sensation or bundle of sensations can contact the mind and deal with the constant emanation of thoughts that is taking place; and by contact (*sparsa*) is meant not merely the surface contact which alone we know out here in our world of superficiality. *Sparsa* or contact is the power of self-identification, the attempt at self-identification of conscious pervasion whereby the self contacts its bodies or whatever it feels itself inclined to be *pro tem*. A conscious thought is not only the resultant of many thought forms as we have said in a previous lesson, but it is also the addition of one more combatant to the world-war, of *Kurukshetra*. The moment a perception in its sevenfoldness is launched into being, a thought or series of thought-forms begins to attack, associate, affect, commingle, resolve, integrate, disintegrate, overpower and make up a result, an event.

Do not fear at all contact with people or with ideas, is the slogan of this lesson. Very true we have asked you not to worry yourself with thoughts that apparently come on to worry you, to cause you fear or make you abandon what you have taken up to do. But the danger here is that students do often avoid the circumstances that give rise to such thoughts, and at the same time do not replace these by other circumstances or surroundings. What we have to understand is to make use (Yoga) of everything of every idea as it comes on to us, at whatever time such idea may come on, provided the idea is not *actually* repugnant or repulsive. The latter require the treatment mentioned in the last lesson; just now we take up ideas born of contact (*sparsa-ja* thoughts).

Let there (*atra*) not (*ma*) be (*astu*) non-contact (*asparsa*) with the thoughts arising from perceptions or percepts. Enjoy everything. These ideas last only their little moment and then pass off; but argue not so to yourself. Do not tell yourself "these ideas, these contacts, their suffering or pain is only momentary, I shall suffer them therefore bravely." That is not the attitude of the Hero or of the Karma Yogi. On the other hand let the attitude be: "These contacts, the suffering and gladness that they are bringing to me, endure mayhap only for the moment; but I shall enjoy them; it is quite possible that another such experience may not at all come in my way in such a fulness, in such a mode, giving such joy, aye such a joy in the suffering. Therefore shall I endure, enjoy, cultivate, intensely conscious, actively and acutely, this experience." Remember herein the self-flagellation of the mystics of the Roman Catholic Church, how intensely they enjoyed pain. You must read Havelock Ellis' book "Psychology of Sex" in six volumes, and if possible the Bibliography referred to therein, especially on *Sader-masoch*. Self-flagellation and pain has its reflex in the disturbance it creates in the sexual sphere; pleasure is but a waste of many useful thought-forms; pain on the other hand provokes many thought-forms into activity that could not otherwise have had any opportunity to manifest itself.

"One's attitude to the necessaries which the traditions of earthly life involve, must of course be to rule them neither by mortification nor by indulgence." Such is the wise rule of *Karma Yoga*; it is not necessary to discard pain just because it is painful, nor is it necessary to revel in pleasant associations. These pleasant associations can only be for their time and it would be only creating a fresh chain of cause-act, (*Karmika*), of event-behaviour were one to attempt to continue the enjoyment. As said already, there happens a separation from the enjoyment, in practice, the separation provokes thought, anger, diversion, and one befogs himself in the attempt. So that when painful thoughts arise in the contacting with objects, all that one has to do is to eliminate mental spines and burrs, to reject or avoid all that one considers inimical to oneself—any attempt to lay down general rules hereunder as to how to do it only leads to confusion, for to each it will be quite different as to what all Ideas are harmful to him. All that one can do at the start to watch, observe, note down (if necessary) consider, study and then reject or eliminate or accept the thought. Probably it sounds all empty literature without definite meaning or precision of message. Wait a bit, however, and listen to us when we tell you to keep a note-book.

It is of course a very small, but it is a very useful hint to keep a note-book beside you as you sit in meditation; after meditation note down any idea or thought that strikes you as strange or curious or out of the ordinary; any idea that you cannot understand; flashes of intuition for which your ordinary thought has not been responsible. Jot down in it all the experiences (thought-forms) that you have had as you sat down to meditation. Write them out in their fullness, especially when they are unique, and keep the book by while you continue your meditations. Not that there is any need to refer to the past pages of the book; rather do not refer back, but just note down your experience and leave it there. The use of the book belongs to another lesson in *Karma Yoga*; what is here taught is that all experiences should be noted especially if they are novel, and dispassionately noted. You can, however, in your leisure hours read over these notes, compare the experience with others in the books in your library if you are an ardent student and can spare time thereto; you can in time understand how much more you learned by suffering them otherwise.

Our point is here that it is by suffering pain, aye, even by courting it, that you can obtain some exquisite sensations of *Karma Yoga*. The Greek philosopher Zeno refers in one of his works to the wise man who having conquered all passions feels happiness in the midst of torture. That is his definition, his ideal of the wise man; the Sanskrit equivalent for which is *Dhira* which also means the Hero. Etymologically it is this way: "Nature, as we know it, is stupid, brutal, cruel, beautiful, extravagant and above all the vehicle of illimitable energy." How do we know it? Only by experience; we realise that the apparent injustice of all differences of well-being can be explained by the fact that we have known prior existences. It is the suffering in this life that has remained and trace back the chain of causes till we got not at a solace but at the only possible conclusion. All suffering then has a meaning and whether the meaning be searched for or not, the suffering should be keenly and intensely enjoyed. The Yogi Philosophy advises the *Karma Yogi* to "work and not to complain—for gradually the state is attained by the *Karma Yogin* where he himself determines the manner in which the impressions of the external world shall affect him."

In most books on *Yoga*, there is far too much emotionalism, not only as part of the language but also as a result of pedantry; the craze for classification has obviously dulled them and they are not able to catalogue experiences, not having had any worth the name. They do give you a long list of the virtues and vices, of the principles and *Tatvas* of the qualifications and *Siddhis* (powers), but as to a correct catalogue of mental experiences on the Path of any *Yoga* you have very few records in plain non-symbolical language. This much remains, that there is apparently no practical attempt to aid suffering, as in the attempt to aid suffering the consciousness of that suffering is lost.

They tell you that *Ahimsa*, non-injury, is the greatest of all virtues, but that greater virtue the cure of those who have undergone *Himsa* is beyond the exoteric schools of Eastern metaphysics. "In order to divide state of thought into 84 classes which is—to their fatuity!—an object in itself because 84 is 7 times 12, they do not hesitate to invent new names for quite imaginary states of the mind and to put down the same state of mind several times." This is what leads to extreme difficulty in the study of their works on Psychology and the like, by the Westerners.

"What we have to remember is that most of the pleasures in life and that of the most education in life are given by superable obstacles. Sport including love, depends on the oncoming of artificial or imaginary resistances. Golf has been defined as trying to knock a little ball into a hole with a set of instruments very ill-adapted for the purpose. In chess, one is bound by purely arbitrary rules." Suffering, I refer to the suffering inflicted by the passing thought as much as to the suffering provoked by contact, is a superable obstacle as is the teaching of the Yogi Philosophy, and the first treatment of suffering is to let it pass. The student is here advised to practise indifference, indifference to any but his own progress. This teaching does not mean the indifference of the Man to the things around him, as it has been often so unworthily and wickedly interpreted. The indifference is a kind of inner indifference; everything is to be enjoyed to the full, everything is to be suffered to the utmost, but always with a reservation that neither shall the absence of the thing enjoyed cause regret nor shall the continuity of the suffering disturb the serenity and patience of the sufferer. May be that this is too hard for the beginner but it is necessary and in many instances it has been found necessary for the beginner to abandon pleasures in order to prove to himself that he is indifferent to them; (An American Brother thinks that it may occasionally be advisable even for the Adept to do this now and again). In the Secret Rules of *Kadambini Diksha,* a very superior kind of Yogic Initiation, it has been ordained on the Yogi that "to succeed he must be fearless, he has to brave danger, death and dishonour, to be forgiving and silent on that which cannot be given; for it is not lawful for an Occultist to thirst or even to seek for revenge." Nay he shall not even say, "Vengeance is Mine, hath said the Lord," to himself.

Such is the ethic of suffering. "The Hindu Yogi has to swear the most solemn oaths never to either desire or seek retaliation or revenge; he has to be always ready to help a brother in danger, even to the risk of his own life; to bury every dead body left unburied; to honor his parents above all; to respect old age and protect those weaker than himself; and finally to ever bear in mind the hour of death and the Purpose that made this body for him." All philosophy is built round suffering; the contemplation of the universe is at first one of pure anguish! The Hindu sees the evil of the environment; the Parsi the *dnij* the permanent enemy of God; in Islam there are *jinn* and devils whom Allah pulls down; in Christianity is the doctrine of original sin to which all are slaves from birth. All these have a moral and the moral is that the suffering and the sin should be borne, understood, fought against. Rest for the Karma Yogi would be unthinkable for it would reduce existence to nothingness. Yes, it is in the travail with the problems of evil that all the great religions of the world have been born.

When the Karma Yogi has started on the programme of life he has sketched for himself, and has a sense of unrest with regard to the environments around him that has deeply entered into his soul there will be no faltering. There will be on the other hand carelessness as to what it may cost the worker himself; he may be crucified or, as it happens in modern days, at the worst, ignored. That is the attitude of the Karma Yogi towards suffering. As says M. Therion: "For to him that is in any wise advanced upon the way of meditation it appears that all objects save one object are dis-

tasteful (blamable) even as appeared formerly
in respect of his chance wishes to the will."
The suffering comes on to him in many ways; dis-
taste, pain, disgust, non-attachment—infliction,
etc. In such cases the most obvious way and a
thorough treatment would be to practise a love of
the suffering, so that "the object is grasped by
the mind and heated in the sevenfold furnace of
love until with explosion of ecstasy they unite
and disappear, for they being imperfect are destroyed utterly in the creation of the perfection of
union." Therion's language is rather hard to
follow but what he says is that the Karma Yogi
should suggest to himself that the suffering he
undergoes is really to be enjoyed, actually to be
longed for, nay to be regretted, if not continued.
The acme of the suffering is to be found only in
the fantastic pain of Bhakti Yoga, Rapture, and
in *Samadhi* where the soul is torn temporarily off
from the body with a sensation as tingling as that
when one's skin is peeled off by oneself.

The test of self-confidence, courage, fortitude,
augmented by bearing sorrow, and disappoint-
ments from the failure of prior undertakings,
with greatness of mind and especially with quiet
and unbroken strength is called the *Agneyi Dhar-
ana,* or *Dhyana Agni, Fire Trial* in the Hindu-
Yogi Philosophy. "All thoughts as they arise
whether on perception or otherwise are subjected

to analysis to an ordeal of their usefulness" to the practitioner irrespective of whatever they are "good or bad." Usefulness is the only test, not whether the Thought is "good" or "bad." We are not concerned with moral judgment at all; rather we would, with Nietsche demand of all philosophers that they have the delusion of the moral judgment beneath them—as there are no such things as moral facts. The danger in moral judgment is that in common with exoteric religion it believes in realities which are not real. Read McSwiney again: "War must be faced, and blood must be shed out gleefully but as a terrible necessity; because there are horrors, moral horrors worse than any physical horror, because freedom must be had at any cost of suffering. The soul is greater than the body. This is the justification for war." Herein do we find the justification for suffering and its use, in this vast untilled field of moral conduct.

Western readers may read H. P. Blavatsky's "Voice of the Silence," that pseudo-Tibetan book, Part II, the Two Paths, verse 23;— "If thou art taught that sin is born of action and bliss of absolute inaction then tell them that they err. Now permanence of human action, deliverance of mind from thraldom by the cessation of sin and fault are not for Deva-Egos . . . (What does H.P.B. mean by Deva-Egos?) . . . Thus saith the doctrine of the Heart . . ." What she says is that one should not be afraid to act; action should be fought by reaction, tyranny will never be overthrown by slavish submission to it; cowardice is conquered by a course of exposing oneself unnecessarily to danger. Suffering has to be enjoyed till it has no effect. "The way to conquer any thought, to overcome any suffering is to understand it and the work of the Karma Yogi herein consists in the ability to decide whether or not he will perform any given action. The Karma Yogi should ever be ready to abide by the toss of a coin and remain perfectly indifferent as to whether it falls head or tail. That is the test of the Karma Yogi, that is the nature of *his* indifference. Be indifferent then to any but thine own work. Thus shall you not be bound."

"Suffer, enjoy every experience as it come on."

SUFFER, ENJOY, EVERYTHING

LESSON VI

We shall now turn our attention to *"Detachment"* which is said to be the meaning of Karma Yoga, and this "detachment" is termed "non-attachment" although the latter phrase conveys no meaning, for the one reason that a negative cannot convey any positive, definite meaning. The difference between the ideas conveyed by *"detachment"* and *"non-attachment"* is that *detachment* is a positive attitude of keeping oneself aloof or detached, while *non-attachment* is vague and of an indefinite meaninglessness which on that account has been made the subject of voluminous commentaries by cheap philosophers to whom we can attribute the desire to legislate for others *via* their public lectures. As says Sankara in his commentary on verse III, 34 of the *Bhagavad Gita*: "Now I shall tell you where lies the scope for personal exertion and for the Teaching (*Sastra*). He who would follow the Teaching should at the very commencement rise above the sway of *affection* and *aversion*. For what we speak of as the nature of a person draws him to its course only through love and aversion. He then neglects his own duties and sets about doing the duties of

others. When on the other hand a person re-
strains these feelings by means of their enemy,
then he will become mindful of the Teaching only
when no longer subject to his own nature. Where-
fore, let none come under the sway of these two;
for they are his adversaries, obstacles to his progress on the right path, like thieves on the road."

The Sanskrit of Sankara is Sanskrit of the 8th
century A. C. and the translator has not expressed
the sense in modern English using philosophical
parlance. What is conveyed is that the practitioner *could* with regard to the objects of objective
world, avoid having either affection or aversion.
He could at all times view the oncoming thought
or contacted object dispassionately; having learned
to let it pass, as stated in Lesson IV, having learned
to bear with it as stated in Lesson V, he might go
a step further and remain quite aloof from it, all
the while eagerly watching the thought fructify
or the object working out the fulfillment.

As already stated, the first position of the Karma Yogin towards the oncoming thought or
towards the universe is to accept it, the next position is to accept it without being affected by it.
The Karma Yogi must especially guard himself
against getting into researches of cosmogony,
against bothering himself as to how the thought
arose, or how it happened. "The question of being is the darkest in all philosophy; all of us are

beggars here; for all of us alike fact forms a
datum, a gift which cannot be burrowed under,
explained away or left behind," says a westerner.
It is as well to leave aside the logical riddle un-
touched of how the coming of whatever it is,
whether it came piecemeal or came it all together
can be or at all logically undersood. In the East
this is termed *Kismet,* the Doctrine of Fatalism in
the form expounded in Islam, of men who have
combined a great sense of personal moral obligation with religious resignation as to the final
outcome of human life. These have been char-
acterized by their meek acceptance of the Present,
of the *Event* as an Act of God, something that
one should not question or trace out; most of the
great religions are clear that life in the world is
a tangle of disharmonies; in one way or another
they say that this world is damned or is the abode
of suffering, but the Doctrine of Kismet says that
these disharmonies are here, this damnation is
here inexplicably. Why indeed explain, ask
they? In the Buddhist metaphysic, the present is
the consequence and the inevitable consequence of
the Past of that Freewill once exercised which
still is available for exercise. The attitude
towards the oncoming Thought must, therefore,
be to put yourself in a proper mental (and physical) condition therefor, to meet it.

Be sane, always. Asceticism is not for you Karma Yogis at all; asceticism excites the mind, the object of the Karma Yogi is not only to calm it but to continue to keep it calm. Of course, during the periods of actual concentration there is no time for any but the work itself, but to make even the mildest asceticism a rule of life is the greatest of errors, except perhaps that of regarding asceticism itself as a virtue. I do not begin here an instruction again asceticism, though asceticism has always been the stumbling block most dreaded by the wise. Christ said that John the Baptist came neither eating nor drinking, and the people called him mad; He himself came eating and drinking and they called him a gluttonous man and a wine bibber and the friend of publicans and sinners. It must always be remembered that the Karma Yogi always does what he likes or rather what he wills and allows nothing to interfere with it, but because he is ascetic in the sense that he has no appetite for the stupidities which fools call pleasure, it has become the fashion with snobs, what we call the *Sastris* of India, to expect him to refuse things both natural and necessary. It has been put to the Karma Yogi that he must accept his environment, and also—wrongly we say—that he should not only accept his environment but also stick on till death to that environment. The notorious caste system had been vainly trying for ages to assert that a cobbler should be a cobbler, an oil-monger an oil-monger, but that only a Brahmin could become a God. Alas, Kabir, Nanak, Chaitanya, and a host of others have been deified and were not Brahmins at all. No doubt the Karma Yogi has no right, no business to break up his domestic circumstances; for the Karma Yogi's doctrine is pat with the Rosicrucian doctrine "that the Adept should be a man of the world, for such is nobler than the hermit."

But under any condition, in every environment, confronted without any proposition or any difficulty, aye, even with destiny in its darkest adversity, it is always open to the Adept to exercise his Freewill. Those who have master souls, says M____, refuse to be bound by anything but their own wills. "They may refrain from certain actions because their main purpose would be interfered with, just as a man refrains from smoking if he is training for a boat-race. But there are sane people so hypercritical that they claim their dislikes as virtue and it very often happens that the literature before the would-be Karma Yogi is full of the self-bombast of the poor, weedy, unhealthy degenerate who cannot smoke because his heart is out of order, and cannot drink because his brain is too weak to stand it or perhaps because the doctor has forbidden him to do it for the next two years, the man afraid of life, afraid to do anything lest some dire result should follow." Very often those acclaimed as the best and greatest of mankind are these slaves to custom and habit those unable to realise that the Karma Yogi must never be *less*, but always *more* than a man. The desire for the flesh has ever grown stronger for ascetics as they endeavoured to combat it by abstinence and when with old age their functions are atrophied they claim vaingloriously "I have conquered," "I have *Vairagya*."

It *is* quite possible to attain *Vairagya*, that sort of indifference that marks a high stage in moral strength; an indifference that approaches disgust for everything—what would remind the Englishman a great deal of the "Oxford manner." It is typically the phlegmatic type which declines to be moved by anything good (bad or indifferent) that does not belong to one. When one is affected by a wrong thought, a thought that does not, however, provoke pain for which latter the treatment has already been given, it is possible for the Karma Yogi to remain indifferent thereto; nay the indifference may be so far strengthend so as to be made a sort of disgust—not expressively so, not even intensively so. The nature of the attitude of disgust herein called *Vairagya* is to remain quite phlegmatic about it, towards undesirable thoughts as towards needless Acts and happenings in the world around the Karma Yogi. Where it is as well to let well alone, it is *the* rule of Karma Yoga to remain indifferent, apparently indifferent all the time. However, the Karma Yogi watches the event, ready to intercede should harm be likely to ensue. The Karma Yogi can remember the famous adage: "Too many cooks spoil the broth —too many physicians kill the patient—too much of care is not necessary about every passing thought."

The attitude of *Vairagya* herein suggested is, of course, a passion-free attitude; there is a particular method open to the Karma Yogi of keeping himself up in the state of equilibrium with which things can be done which bear no fruit and have no reaction. The Eastern Scriptures state that the Yarma Yogin's status is like that of fishes in water, of kites in the air; they affect not the element in which they move. The Karma Yogi lives and moves in the world but he lives and moves practically incognito, practically as if he were mking himself invisible, while continuing to work. It is best to explain this attitude by a praxis which has been advised and I quote the advice at length:

> The student must set aside a small part of his daily life in which to concern himself with something quite different from the objects of his daily occupation. (Five minutes a day will suffice.)
> He is not to occupy himself with the affairs of his own ego or with the thoughts that occur to

him, in such moments. He should rather let the thoughts he experiences as messages from the outer world re-echo within his own completely silent self. (And note, you, yourself have to be *utterly* silent, the silence being assured by your taking up the attitude of disgust—*Vairagya*.)

N. B.—And he will prepare himself to receive quite new impressions of the outer world through different eyes. (He need not be waiting particular results at all; he ought not to do so.)

For it is quite possible to view the universe through various kinds of spectacles, from various points of view; and similarly it is possible to consider each oncoming thought from a different point of view. The hint is to change your Point of View rather than attempt to change the Thought by going into the whence and why of it. He may of course remain perfectly indifferent to the experience furnished by the Thought, and the reason for the indifference requires to be better understood.

Just as the seven forms of perception and contact by perception generate a sevenfoldness of thought, so every thought deals with seven planes of experience in eastern psychology as stated by the *Vedas*. They are: (1) Memory, *Smriti*, (2) Vision, *Pratyaksha*, (3) Association, *Aitihya*, (4) Induction, *Anumana*. These four planes of thought work in collaboration and interrelation

with thoughts from (5) the *Sanchita,* the store-
house that is the individual make-up; (6) Association or contact with which creates another
thought, *Prarabda;* (7) accidental sympathetics,
Agamya, crowning the whole. When the attention
runs as a shuttle does through this warp it creates
a weft of Action and Reaction called *Samsara.*
One way to avoid this creation of *Samsara* is to
deal with the original thought and inhibit it, by
remaining in an attitude of disgust theretowards,
and the attitude of disgust or *Vairagya* has to be
taken up to every thought other than the subject of
meditation. And before the attitude of disgust
should the attitude of watchfulness hereinbefore
advised be taken up.

All that is required in this stage is an inhibition
of thought. The Karma Yogi has to recognise
that the thought that occurs to him is very necessary in itself and ought to be borne with, suffered,
allowed to pass on without regard to any end outside itself. This thought as has been mentioned is
but a resultant, a reaction and hence cannot be
avoided. But at the same time it is very necessary to avoid treating the thought as an actuality
or reality. To do so is a further action, a further-
ance of "bondage," as has already been said. It
may even be necessary to put oneself in an attitude of disgust. A little later the practice of
elimination of thoughts could be tried, but so far

the neophyte Karma Yogi has to train himself to
change his point of view, whenever he has to deal
with an experience that is alien to his own will. He,
as it were, goes up the "Hill of Meditation," take
up a point of view of *Udaseenata*, a sort of view
of the plains as from the top of a hill, a compre-
hensive view, the view of a superior person. How
can the Karma Yogi think as a God, if he has not
the outlook of a God, the *Isvara Bhava*! And to
have the outlook of a God one has to change his
own point of view, the point of view that is as but
putty in the hands of Intelligence. Towards the
on-coming thought what the Karma Yogi here
has to do is to judge for himself whether to God
such a thought would be possible, before he en-
tertains the thought. This *Isvara Bhava* has also
been spoken of as the attitude of the *Kshatriya*,
Kshatra denoting both the Kingdom of God and
the Human Body (soul and body combined).
Just as nothing can exonerate the Karma Yogi
from doing his utmost to determine and perform
the right Act and just as nothing can excuse his
failure to do so, in the plane of thought "culture"
(miscalled), nothing can exonerate the Karma
Yogi's failure to obtain the right thought by the
process hereinbefore mentioned.

But if these themselves were not enough, a
settled practice has been encouraged by the Hindu-
Yogi Philosophy with regard to wrong thoughts—

namely to eliminate them. The charge to the Karma Yogi has always been to eliminate rubbish from the Mind—he should eliminate anything which does not serve his purpose. He can, as by the *"Neti," "Neti" mantra* eliminate (and thus select for use) thoughts pouring in as he sits to meditation. As each thought comes on before you, you, having been trained already by the practices before mentioned and not being the slave of the thoughts, being careless about the results, begin by examining the thought and reject it, if you think it useless to yourself, by the Mantra *"Neti,"* Not so; *"Neti,"* Not thus; Oh, no, certainly not. This *"Neti," "Neti"* process requires a very deep psychological investigation as a preliminary. It is not sufficient to get rid temporarily of these thoughts; one must as it were seek their roots and destroy their roots so that they can never rise again. A helpful suggestion is to bring about the habit by auto-suggestion of declining thoughts that are not useful to one's purpose, as a settled practice of Karma Yoga by the use of the Mantra

"NETI, NETI"

All along you have to remember that your experiences, (again these thoughts that you are advised to deal with) are not the ultimate truth. They are only sensations that change with your status and as you advance in the direction of more and more untiring energy. "Thine to do" is with thought only, says the Bhagavad Gita; "not with the results"—which results are the resultants of the whole universe acting on the Act initiated perhaps by you, the reaction of your action. It is quite open to you, Karma Yogi, to take out use for anything into yourself—because yours is the kingdom of thought—but it is as well that you do not revel in the silence of not dealing with the occurring event, as it or as you require. This carelessness as to what it may cost the Karma Yogin is to be found more in the West nowadays apparently combined with the desire and impulse to work; and if it is not to be found in the East, it is because the conditions of life possible in the *Sannyasi* mode of living have made it unnecessary for anyone to be a Karma Yogin at all. And the commingling of the West and East have made it equally impossible for a *Grihee* (householder) to be a Yogi, much less a Karma Yogin unless he be truly ardent.

NA ITI NA ITI

NOT THUS, NOT THIS

LESSON VII

We propose now to take up a section of Karma Yoga that has been rejected or rather misunderstood, namely the use of sacraments to the Karma Yogi. It had been an invariable statement by religious reformers that in spite of the inferiority of Vedic ritual still it had its uses. What the uses are to the Karma Yogi has not been explained but it has been taken that Karma Yoga (of the lower or inferior (?) variety) consisted in the observance of the Vedic ritual and performances of the practices mentioned in the *Vedas*. For there is much in the *Vedas* that is of use in magic, in religion, in praxis, though great be the difficulty in cogent arrangement, and greater the worry on the part of the Teacher not to speak overmuch; lest in unlocking Pandora's box disease and devilment get out to work their havoc with simple minds anxious to use every good advice as a weapon against one's neighbour. Great indeed are our difficulties and nothing but the desire to help humanity on the part of the Latent Light Culture has compelled me to write down what little I am permitted to do. Alas, I am not complete; I would rather request that if difficulties crop up, and difficulties will crop up only to the evil-minded, aye, even if a single thought of evil be encouraged, the reader addresses the Latent Light Culture for remedy.

First then as to the rationale of the *Karma Kanda,* religious ritual. It is very necessary that the rationale be understood first before the subject is approached. To begin at the beginning we would draw attention to our original statement that the universe is a universe of Thought. Herein we venture to state that it is *naught* else. All objects are but thoughts, whether we see them as *Behaviours* or feel them as *sensations* or do not see them at all as thoughts. Thought is a constant function irrespective of the Ego, of you or I; the universe is a play of strands of thought working out among other strands of thought and what marks out each strand (*guna*) of Thought (*Karma*) is an Event of Time, the fourth dimension. Just as the geometrical point in space is a line or thread of event in space—Time the 4th dimension, each event is but the occurrence of a Thought, a tick mark placed on thought which is matter of the 5th dimension; for Thought transcends and is irrespective of Time. From the viewpoint of Time, Thought is *Immortal,* or rather *beyond* Time. Thought does not age, has neither **Past,** Present nor Future and always can be recalled—though not in the same form or vehicle in which it first appeared. This is the first Truth about Thought.

Secondly, from the viewpoint of the Thinker, the Mind or what emanates Thoughts, what is behind Thought, what of which Thought is but an Image or debased image, Thought is a *Sacrifice*, *Yajna*. This is a most Sacred Truth. It is another way of stating that each Thought having been emanated returns (by the Law of Action and Reaction) back to the Thinker, *Mind* (*Brahma*). But the emanation and the return are *not* meaningless at all; a thought is *not* a waste; a Thought is a *Purposeful* emanation and returns with its *Purpose* fulfilled; this is not an assertion but a matter of experience (*Anna*). It is *for* the experience that Thought comes to be (*Bhoota*); it is *from* out of experience (*Anna*) that the Thought that has come to be, has been made, and gathering unto Itself the experience it gains, the Thought (Son) returns to his Father (Mind) which art in Heaven When therefore God created mankind, says Genesis I.28, "And God said unto them (and God blessed them)—Be fruitful and multiply . . . . replenish the earth and subdue it": Exactly what the *Bhagavad Gita* says (III, 10): "God the Lord of Progeny having created Progeny (*Praja*) along with sacrifices (*Yajna*) said of old, before creation, Hereby do you multiply. These shall be the ful-

fillers of your desires," or words to that effect.
Of course the progeny were thoughts and each
thought was an Act of Sacrifice or an Act of Worship of God (or of God's command or Act). Mind
you, they, the thoughts, were to be fulfillers of
themselves, of their desires, their own milkmaids
for themselves the milch cows. As says the
proverb, why have of the Kingdom of the Mind
half the kingdom; have the whole of course.

Each thought is of the Form of Light—a *Devata*—but yet each thought is still helpless, the
phrase *Deva* conveys the idea of helplessness also.
Each *Devata* (Thought) as created, when it goes
to the make-up of your Being, has virtually all
the qualities of the cell-life (in the human body).
Just as you have to understand the capacity of the
subsconscious cell life in you, that builds and re-
builds your body, so must you understand the
power of these Thoughts emanated by you or by
mankind. Filling the atmosphere round about
you are Thoughts, Intuitive messengers, Mr.
Stillwell in his book "Grow and Live Young" calls
them. "Expect them, command your intuitions
to come to your aid when problems confront you;
consider that Intuition is a silent partner, that it
desires to aid and will aid if called on for help."
And the *Bhagavad Gita* says equally well: "Consider then each cell of your body, each psycho-
mere (particle of your soul) has ears and be care-

ful what is whispered by your Thoughts and Acts, into these ears, what you tell your subconscious, for whatever the order is, the cell will build *you* up accordingly. Have ye not noted that sudden psalms of fear or anger kill like lightning? We would go further and say: "Be careful what thought you add on to the *world of thoughts*— for they both mar and make—unerringly."

Very curious this our suggestion—it is Vedic— that thought is a sacrifice, and as a sacrifice a rite whereby not only man gains divine help but the Gods themselves derive strength, a means by which man assists Gods against evil. This was the teaching in the ancient Parsi country. The existence of angels and devils has been part of the religious literature of almost all countries; in one form or another; and what are these angels or devils but the visions of Thoughts embodied? All along has prevailed the idea that the function of men was to strengthen the Gods (Thoughts) by Prayer (persistent Thought) and Sacrifice (more Thought). Among the Parsis the teaching was that if Gods were not pleased or sacrificed to they hurt humanity; so too among the Hindus where the Pitris the manes of dead ancestors have similarly to be appeased; and in China and Japan where ancestor worship was the only worship— the ancestor being ourselves! In Sanskrit *Mata* (Mother) was a synonym for *Atma* which meant father and son equally well—being too reflexive a pronoun. Indeed there is much in the ancestor worship of ancient nations to be understood and appreciated in the light of our philosophy today and only a portion of the entire truth need be considered now.

As said already, on the earth nearly a hundred thousand persons die every day, the great majority of which are unconscious, purposeless monads—the atmosphere is full of them. They remain for some time in the atmosphere, disperse and form a cosmic environment of diffused consciousness which mingles with the "subconscious" at times and manifests in mediumistic and spiritistic phenomena. This leads us to a brief study of Death and what happens at "death"— and in the state beyond Death. We of course do not take up the materialistic theory that Death is a mere disruption of the congregation of the cells called the body which congregation breaks up leaving the cells free to form other congregations somehow. Such a theory is not for thinkers, not for Karma Yogis to whom every Act in Nature has a meaning, to whom Death is a conscious, voluntary act and not an incident. Death is a "laying aside" of the outer-shell which has become independent of the directing Thought—called "Soul" or Spirit—death is the death of the shell, an act of anarchy on the part of the cells composing the shell, these cells having chalked out a course against or independently of the soul.

What happens at death then? Fournier D'Albe puts it in his excellent language: "A nucleus weighs about 1/1000th of the average cell body; its really vital and perhaps invisible portion may be 1/10000th part of the weight of the nucleus. In other words taking all the cells together, our real living matter, the vital portions of the body may have an aggregate weight of about 1/5th of an ounce. Could we eliminate all the rest of the cell material we should have a body consisting of all that is alive in every single cell. But (especially note this) that body would be quite invisible and would if it filled the outline of the body as before ascend some fifteen miles in the air before it found a position of equilibrium. It could indeed live in a new world, retaining all its social and organic memories and fulfilling all its essential conditions except that of acting on ponderable matter." It will be enough to say that at death, the soul, itself a "body" composed of all that is vital in every cell is "released" and soars to the upper atmosphere.

To us the soul is not a mere "cloud" of physical (albeit fine) inert matter. It is a Life, a Purpose, the unfulfilled portions of the Purposes that animated the late dead body; a Purpose all the more strong because it had been rid of the clog that was recently hampering it. And to confirm this comes in the statements of the earnest band of thinkers and workers who from messages, codified messages for which the vehicle-body was not responsible, which say that the invariable assertion from the realms beyond Death is that the conditions on the other side of Death are much like those here more than the communicators (the recent dead or disembodied) themselves had expected; that the character and personality are unchanged; but that they are freer from obstruction and difficulty and that the conditions are more conducive to progress than here; and at the same time they assure us that they know little more than we know, that they have not suddenly jumped into supernal or infernal regions at all. Indeed it would appear that the dead here around us, through us, in us (?), and that they are connected in their plane by links of affection and interest rather than space relation or bodily proximity. None the less the dead are barely cognisant of earth happenings, curiously.

Another and outstanding fact in early messages is the keen desire apparently felt to relieve the minds of survivors of some anxiety or misunderstanding which is casting a shadow over their lives; for the Dead are as we said, but unfulfilled Purposes and as such deserving of the sympathy and worship of those on this side of the veil. For the very best thinkers, like Mahomed Rasul Allah (Peace Be on Him), have opined that "the development of a man's faculties is really the starting point towards an immeasurable wider vista of the realms to be traversed opening out after death when the soul is liberated and assumes another body in Paradise in accordance with past deeds; similarly those who have wasted their opportunity in this life shall under the law which makes every man taste of what he has done be subjected to a course of treatment till the effect of their poisonings be nullified after which they are fit again to start on to the great goal, God's Mercy." This in the language of the spiritualists is expressed in the following quotation: "The same constructive ability as must in the long course of evolution have succeeded in producing the visible organism by arranging particles of matter seems able to continue its task under the new conditions and can construct another new body or mode of manifestation out of such substance as is there available; the ether it may hypothetically be supposed to be, a body not unlike the body it had here."

Writing on the exteriorisation of personality, Fournier D'Albe says that "the observed stability of our body, its constancy of outline, is due to the play of imponderable forces vast in comparison with the size of the particles on which they act.

On this view this body is a kind of *mist* from which there is a possibility of extracting a finer kind of mist and doing so in a short time and repeatedly with a nearly permanent possibility of restoring it to its former place; and this is herein significant that the force of cohesion which keeps the body together is almost certainly of electrostatic origin."

We can understand this better when we recognise that man is but an aggregation of many thoughts each thought a *mist*; the dead are only the mist separated from the body, but the term *mist* must not be understood an unity but rather a multiplicity of very unstable composition, and, look you, a multiplicity that *still* grows, decays, reforms, continues to be of the same material, namely, of *thoughts*. Not all these thoughts are forms; many are inchoate, they are incomplete in form; others are mere velocities, powers, yearnings, what the *Bhagavad Gita* calls in its language, Fires, Flames, Radiances, smokes, nights, luminosities, months, days, blacknesses, to denote the denizens of the realms beyond death of the physical.

Free intercourse with the realms of the dead was possible and is still possible; experiments continually being made by spiritualists are proving the possibility. Whether such free intercourse and intermingling of the living with the dead is advisable is more than the Hindu scriptures can say. Writing on the reappearances of the forms of the dead, a gifted author says: "The subjective form created through the desires and thoughts in connection with things of matter survives the death of the body; the pale copy of the man that was, his eidola, vegetates for a period of time but will, if left to itself, gradually fade out and disintegrate. Occasionally, however, these reclothe themselves out of the materials at hand which are found in the air and in the emanations of those present at seances and then become objective; but ordinarily they do not perceive us nor we them. But it is sinful to recall them, sinful to retard their progress by worrying them to repeat their past here."

According to the *Rg Veda* the dead go to that joy that Yama the pioneer discovered for them; a passage in the *Shatapatha Brahamana* XI.4.iv.2 says that the dead live in intercourse with *Brahma* (God). How then arose the idea of the rites to the *manes,* the rites other than mere invocations or worship? On which states the Buddhist: "The unsatisfied desire of beings that belong to a state of personal existence in the material world has a force, has creative impulse in itself so strong that it attracts as center a new Purpose drawing God back again to mundane life." We here tread on the theory of *reincarnation,* a theory that has *not* been accepted in the earlier writings and even where accepted has been considered to be optional and never compulsory as in latter writings.

The suggestion herein is that Thought can become dominant, can survive death, can rebuild again a body, can after death affect the world that it got out of; the suggestion is that such thoughts *have* to be treated with by the Karma Yogi, for the teaching is that such dominant Thoughts of the dead do seek help and punish us in the world if neglected. Hence the rites to the dead, the *Pitr Kriyas*, to the *Fravshi* of the Parsis. Incidentally, reflection would lead to a greater understanding of the universe of thought as existing beyond Time and circumstance (body).

All worship, all sacrifice, all religion began as has been seen in the History of Religions with the worship of the dead, either as our ancestors or as heroes or as sages; in China worship has been and is offered only to the ancestors; in the Turanian countries to the dead who have been interred in *Samadhi* (tombs or temples) and who are still living; in Egypt to the "dead" Pharaohs whose mummies reposed in pyramids, in undisturbed peace; in among the Aryas to the Pitrs, the father and mother, chiefly; for, as has been stated, it is not only now but for ever so long a time that the dead have become immortal memories for the dying who remained.

In the Indian doctrine, the dead have to be pleased by what has now become a small offering of sesame seeds (*thila*) and rice (*akshatah*) along with water in an act called *tarpana* (for pleasing). Almost all adult-males are to be found after their fathers' death offering this every New Moon day, after mid-day, to the ancestors and this rite called *Pitr Kriya*, of all the ordained rites, still survives other rites and hence is taken up for explanation.

Thilah stand for all the best that is in man, the best of his good thoughts, the best of his *yogaic* practices; as has been said the dead are not merely the personalities that were, but only fragments thereof; they are the still-to-be-fructified purposes and thoughts, good, bad, and indifferent that were of a deceased personality but now are disintegrating, or are remaking, or getting along, in another world that is still linked to us by ties of affection, each one fragment a make-up of thoughts that *do* form our thought environment. It is still, in this age too, seen from messages from beyond the veil that there are desires, there too, to communicate with us here and to make us respond; and the only way to establish such communication is *via* the *thought* world; good thoughts (*thila*), undying memories (*akshatas*) are to be sent up along with the desire to please (*Tarpana*). The "form" for the act is the offer of the sesame seeds and rice grains along with water, of which a handful; if the dead are those who have become recluses, the offering was of pure milk alone; for such did not want solace but mere kind remembrance, if at all. Yet, the Karma Yogi ought, of course, to remember the dead who have fed, who have inspired, who have educated us and are still doing so. What form this ancestor worship, as you may call it, *should* take depends on the metaphysic of the worshipper; on his spirituality rather, for in the act he is outpouring his self on in sacrifice, in the sacrifice of what is called *"Pitr Yajna."* In India this outpouring consists in feeding all and sundry relations and poor of the same caste on the anniversary day of the death of the deceased object; and this is actually soliciting the good thoughts of the many fed towards what remains of the old personality of the dead. And the ritual combines also the offer to the ancestors of the oblations of cooked rice and ghee into the Fire, specially invoked and consecrated by magick, as per tradition-honored ritual. Thoughts here are offered in generous sacrifice, (*ahuti*) in their collective (*pinda*) to the ancestors; to the ancestors; fire and water the destroyers and solvents of all things (actually they are the transmuters of thoughts from the inchoate to the actual)—are asked to help in a generous conveyance of the good thoughts from man to what was man.

We think that the West does require some sort
of rites to the dead other than "in memorium"
masses for the soul and the keeping up the anniversary day of great men. We think that especially in spiritualist circles there should be greater
consideration shown to the dead. All invocations
should be made of the dead with *reverence*; the
spirits called up should be assured that they are
called up for *their own sake* primarily; is there
any purpose remaining unfulfilled for them, is
there anything we, the living, can do to meet the
unfulfilled wishes of the dead we invoke?   As
they sit in silent circles in the dark, this may be
the attitude of the enquirers, and such an attitude
will remove much of the stigma that is gradually
sullying the good work done by the spiritualists.

Whether the Western Karma Yogin should
adopt the entire Hindu rituals of the dead *Srardhas*
(anniversary rituals) is another matter; what we
can state is that the additional charity of the offer
of free food to the poor on anniversary days will
not be a wrong act anywhere in the world; nor will
the Hindu injunction to regard anniversary days
as holy like unto the Sabbath be without value for
adoption. But the puzzle is that Occidentals (to
whom the personality of the dead remains unchanged) have no rites for the dead of an anniversary ritual nature whereas the Orientals, who
believe in the change of the personality after

death, continue to behave as if the personality had been continuing on unchanged even after death.

LESSON VIII

The Hindu-Yogi Philosophy has recognised full well the universe of Thought in so far as to state that Thoughts people many realms of existence beyond the physical plane, the treatment of one of which we have already spoken of in the last chapter. Thoughts exist otherwise too, as the denizens, for instance, of the infra world, the matter of biology, for which the term in Hindu philosophy is *Bhoota* (what has come to be); as ideas, soul particles, psychomeres, gods, divinities, angels, good thoughts, *Devas*, denizen of a supra world, (not superior world at all); as *Manushyas*; men themselves who are but aggregations of Thought; and as the Transcendentals, the Higher Purposes of Man called in the collective God. The Karma Yogi has to know, has to appreciate these lives, these Thoughts as forming part of the universe he is dealing with, and has to settle his attitude towards these various forms of thought not as they come before him, but collectively, comprehensively.

As he can approach the *Devas*, the gods of the supra world, and help the *Bhootas*, the beings of the infra world, alike *via* the agency of Fire, says *Veda*. And by fire is meant not merely the flame but the catalyst that accelerates oxidation, which oxidation is a constant ceaseless factor in the universe, the same thing again as thought. We shall therefore deal with the Fire mystery, for Fire is a mystery, as great a mystery as catalysis, as great a mystery as electrical induction, as radiography; Fire has been a universal symbol; it was the universal medium for all offerings among almost all the ancient nations. And has the use and purpose of fire been entirely meaningless? The Karma Yogi must understand why the ancient Parsis and Hindus were charged with being worshippers of the visible fire, *and falsely charged, too.* For the Parsis and Hindus face the Fire as they also face the sun and sea, because in them they picture to themselves the hidden light of lights, source of all life, to which they give the name of Ahuramazda. How well Robert Fludd, the English mystic, expresses this divinity of Fire is seen from the following excerpt from "Hargrave Jennings on the Rosicrucians," p. 69.

"Regard fire then with other eyes than with those soulless incurious ones with which thou hast lookt on it as the most ordinary thing. Thou has forgotten what it is, or rather thou hast never known. Chemists are silent about it. Philosophers talk about it as anatomists talk about the constitution or parts of the human body. It is made for man and the world and it is greatly like him they would add that is *mean.* . . . But is this all? Is this the sum of the casketed lamp of the human body? thine own body, thou unthinking world's machine, thou man? Or in the fabric of this clay lamp (what a beautiful simile) burneth there not a light? Describe that ye doctors of physics! Note the goings of fire . . . . Think that this thing is bound up in matter chains. Think that he is outside of all things; and that thou and that world are only the thing between and that outside and inside are both identical, couldst thou understand the supernatural truth! Reverence fire for its meaning and tremble at it. Avert the face from it as the Magi turned, dreading and as the symbol bowed askance. . . . Wonder no longer then if, rejected so long as an idolatry, the ancient Persians and their masters the Magi concluding that they saw all in this supernaturally magnificent element, fell down and worshipped it; making of it the physical representation of the very truest yet in man's speculation and in his philosophies—nay in his commonest reason impossible God."

And look you, this is the language not of a Parsi or Hindu but of an English scholar, one of a nation of phlegmatics, and hence is his effusiveness remarkable; of one who followed the shining path marked out by the Chaldean Magi and obtained like them the true meaning of their mysteries.

Fire (*Agni*) was not merely a symbol with the ancient Hindus; it was a vehicle for the good thoughts of the individual and good thoughts were offered up along with material physical offerings *via Agni* the great Vehicle, *vahana*. Could not good thoughts, kind wishes and the like be offered without any media? They could, of course, but they would in most cases be inchoate; of incomplete cogency, and hence ineffective of action. But offering through Fire conveys to the offerer the suggestion that the *Vedas* state about the Vedic sacrifices; namely that offerings into the fire being reduced all into one element rise up to the Father the Sun who himself is a great drier of water which rises in steam up to him; from on high where these smokes and clouds form and in time condense cometh rain which sheds on the world forcing up plant life and creating fruits which are offered again in sacrifice. As says the ancient lawgiver Manu: "The offering put into the fire goeth to the Sun; from the Sun cometh rain; from rain food; from food all creatures." III. 76.

And again, as says *Ramanuja*, a great revivalist of Hindu Bhakti Yoga in his comment on the *Bhagavad Gita* III. 15: "Thus is the wheel of ceaseless antecedents and sequences, thus; food from rain, rain from *yajna*, sacrifice and worship; *yajna* from works performed by a doer; works from a living body; living bodies again from food."

The world is seen by the ancient Vedic yogis to be a world of fire, of things which are *ceaselessly* burnt up; what the chemists mean when they say that oxidation is a constant process of nature; what the ancient works state when they say that Thought is a constant process irrespective of any thinker; what the Xian mystics mean when they say that the world is a world of sin that has been already saved by the sacrifice of Jesus Christ who is dying on the Cross in every moment of time. All things are being burnt up, eaten up, continuously and it is for the Karma Yogi to make of this unconscious *waste* process a useful process, to regulate it, to make all thoughts, offerings, to render the thought again to its appropriate end. And herein is Fire to be used as apparatus (*vahana*), water as an accessory (*tarpana*), and speech as the time marker, rhythm fixer (*japa*); for the Karma Yogi is going to use all the material available and use it for the ends of all, ends that are to be attained in the universe as far as he can help. And let not this programme daunt any one, for the one instrument that he Karma Yogi shall use is good thought, and if he uses it, he does not care about what happens in the use, especially to himself, and of course he does not care about the results at all.

The rationale of the burnt offering is this: That the offering is reduced to aerial particles according to science and as all particles are ions of ether (or fine matter), if you please, the burnt offering is reduced to a diffused condition just as the thought world is, and as we have postulated the thought world is a world of matter still, albeit finer matter than any we have out here; for thought can be used, rejected, eliminated, placed, transmitted, avoided, rendered up just as any other material can be. And along with the burnt offering goeth the prayer or persistent thought of the offerer, goeth up to the object intended much quicker than the offering itself, for who can state that the offering as reduced in fire has not reached the object; who can say that the object of affection did not exist *in* the Fire and did not take the offering as it was offered to the Fire? And indeed fire itself is but a form of thought, a form of oxidation, a form of Life.

In the Turanian worship, the worship *via* fire and the burnt offering were replaced by the offer of incense; good thoughts, kind remembrances and the like expressions of gratitude were offered up in incense, frankincense and spices, the smoke of which added to the world's greater fragrance. The Turanian concept did not need the sacrifice of the fire; it ruled that man should sacrifice himself by a willing life and by a willing death; but in effect

they offered good thoughts to the universe of
thoughts by the burning of incense, itself provo-
cative of fragrant thoughts. The Western World
has virtually adopted the Turanian ritual; it
maintains the offer of incense still and has given
up the burnt offering and any attempt to intro-
duce the burnt offering in the West would be difficult; what we would therefore advise is that
every Karma Yogi, every disciple who has come to
us for guidance, do, in a separate room set apart
for worship, meditation or Yoga as it ought to be,
burn incense or joss sticks, as the Chinese or Jap-
anese do; incense of any non-stupefying kind, before his invocation of the Presences around and in
man, before beginning each practice of meditation.
It would be very well if along with this offer
of incense, good wishes for the welfare of the
world around, be also sent up by the use of any
short prayer, such as the *"Phala-sruti-vakyas"* of
Sanskrit books for the Orientals, or the simpler
"Sarvey janah sukhinah bhavantu," "let every
one be happy; let every one have his peace," "the
Blessings of Alla on all"—any of these may be
adopted for use as *mantra* or affirmation.

For Orientals and for those Karma Yogins of
the West who have a liking for Oriental methods,
it is advisable to have an *altar*; in the West where
tables and chairs are used the altar has to be
raised and all that one has to do is to have such a

separate altar for himself, instead of the common altar at church or lodge. Of course the altar should be used exclusively for the purpose of the Ritual and be kept clean and pure. Every morn after one has risen and finished his morning ablutions and cleansing, his bath and dressing (of course the loose morning gown is enough) one may offer to the fire that he has kindled, (it is only a little flame of burning scented wood sticks, the scent being all important), a handful of cooked wheat or rice or oats seasoned with butter or aromatic oil, or a few scented sticks of wood along with the repetition of that grand hymn, Our Lord's Prayer.

Such of our Mahomeddan Karma Yogis as desire to take up the hint contained in the above may, instead of the above Prayer, repeat the *Fateha*, a very ancient Tamil Prayer rendered into the Arabic, and drop the fire offering, keeping on the burning of the incense.

Those who would have no objection to the Hindu ritual are required to offer two offerings, first to our Father the Sun, *Sooryaya Svaha*; and next to Fire the great granter of one's yearnings, good yearnings (of course), *Agnaye Su Ishta kritaya svaha.* It is taken that the place of fire-kindling, the altar, has been well cleansed and that Fire is approached with reverence; the Parsis say that the mouth must be covered by a veil lest any spittal, or even the breath, pollute the Fire addressed. These are the essentials and may be used with any adaptation required by modernity with the proviso that neither flesh, fish, blood nor foul-smelling substances be used in the ritual; and it will be a pleasing diversion to many westerners to adopt this mode of prayer and offering.

The ancient Hindu identified Fire with himself, with his household life (*garhapatya*), with his service to humanity and the world (*ahavaniya*), with the invocation of the Higher presence (in himself and in the universe), *darsana*. There were kept, first one fire that was ever burning, and next three fires, two of them periodical, or occasional. The Hindu recognised the Fire in man, Hunger, *Agni Vaisvanara*, God in himself, the living God in man that we all recognise in our acceptance of charity as a virtue. God has incarnated as man with a Purpose, wherefor is the body, we have to live to fulfill the Purpose (*Anta*), and we have to eat to live, not because it is the food that causes the vital energy, but because vital energy, oxidation or thought, a constant process, has been eating up the matter-cells that we have to replace to make our embodiment hold together. God himself as *Agni* (fire) *Vaisvanara* (in all men) digests and converts gross material into experience, both mental, spiritual and physical.

As says the Westerner, "the satisfaction afforded by a starving creature by his taking food is a mani-

festation of the spirit, of the spirit of God in man,"
that is where the rationale of Charity comes in as
a *Manushya Yajna,* sacrifice to and worship of
humanity. In Mahommeddanism, Charity was
the one injunction of duty from man to man and
was regarded as a duty to be controlled and regu-
lated by the state; in the Hindu country the offer
of food to the guest was a duty to be well recognised; for here the guest was God himself and
the unhonored guest took away the merit of the
host. It was to be regarded, say the Hindu scriptures, that the unbidden guest was a messenger of
God, one whom God could not feed and hence
whom God had sent to us to be fed, fed as *God*
should have fed him, for it was God's duty to feed
every creature. Not one shall die of starvation say
the scriptures; the sun shall not set before every
one is fed; the great creator, *Brahma* himself,
shall feed the starving.

The Karma Yogi (like every householder)
should satisfy, recognising their needs, all beings
on all the five planes where worship or sacrifice is
to be rendered. Firstly then as to the human
plane, charity the offer of free food to the chance
guest, to the really needy as much as any one could
afford, has been advised in Hinduism and Jainism. Hindu scriptures have gone elaborately on
this duty to the needy, of giving food, to the ex-
tent that it has been made part of the ordinances

that none was to take food unless he had fed
strangers seeking food at his doorstep; but before
feeding strangers the householder had to feed
children, vestals, sick females, aged females, aye,
before feeding even the guest! So much was the
guest esteemed in the East that the guest was regarded as the master of the house, even before the
master himself. The ancient adage also states
that the housholder attains heaven not so much
by sacrifices, or charities or by attendance on the
Fire, as by devotion to the unbidden guest.

Not only was man to be fed by the householder but also the lives in the "infra" world, the
teeming life of the insect world as far as possible
in what is known as the *Bhoota Yajna* by offerings
called *Bali*. Like *Devas*, the beings of the infra
world can hardly be seen and hence the offer of
food to them must be through the medium of the
elements (in this case the elements of air and
earth); food is spread or scattered before the birds,
ant or insect life, snakes even, in groves, nocturnal
wanderers in midnight offerings, of food and
drink where four roads meet, or in cemeteries.
Along with the offer of the food go out the good
thoughts of the offerer of the food, thoughts that
go out to strengthen the *Bhootas,* the beings of the
lesser world that is of us, that is contributing its
quota to us. It *was* useful in ancient time to offer
blood periodically to one class of these beings and

in many places blood continues to be shed and
offered in the invocation of the beings of the infra
world. *Bali* was current in very ancient time
among the Turanians and consisted in the offer of
the blood and flesh of the sacrificed animal victims
to insect and bird life, the while the sacrifice was
considered as an offering to God, i.e. to the Being
to be pleased or appeased.

Dating to very ancient times when the victim
was God or one deified as God for the purpose of
the immolation, as in the *Purusha Sukta, Aja
Medha*, etc., of the *Rg Veda*, it came out later on
that instead of a human victim an animal victim
representative of God was sacrificed to God in a
hundred fashions in many thousand primitive
cults. "Sacrifice to gods," says James (*Varieties of
Religious Experience*), "are omnipresent in prime-
val worship, but as cults have grown refined,
burnt offerings and the blood of he-goats have
been superseded by sacrifices more spiritual in nature; Judaism, Islam and Buddhism get along
without ritual sacrifice, so does Christianity, save
in so far as the notion is preserved in transfigured
form in the mystery of Christ's atonement."

Says Madame H. P. Blavatsky in her *Isis Un-
veiled*, II. 41: "As an expiation for the past, present and future sins of ignorant but nevertheless
polluted mankind the Hierophant (Karma
Yogi) had the option of suffering his sinless life

as the sacrifice for his race to the Gods whom he
hoped to rejoin or an animal victim (Passion).
The former depended entirely on his free will."
Like Jesus the Karma Yogi's life is one of voluntary sacrifice, for it is not as a halter that he regards (his duties) these rituals nor as helping *him*
on, but because they are God's work. To the idea
of charity as the virtue to be practised towards
man, the Karma Yogi adds that all shedding of
blood, all use of flesh and fish as food should be
accompanied by the recognition of the need of
the poor, too poor to buy the food, a fact that
Islam recognises and insists on to be appreciated
in the course of the Haj pilgrimage.   It has, it
may be mentioned *en passant*, been part of Hindu
ethics to spread food for crows, birds, insects, etc.,
the *Bhootas,* before beginning the daily meal;
whether this can be followed out in the West is
a matter of individual choice, but is it after all
anything worse than feeding the pigeons or mag-
pies, than feeding dogs and horses?

So far as to *Bhoota Yajna*; but what about the
milliards of beings in himself, what about his
higher purposes? We have seen how in the history
of religious thought, religions such as Islam,
Christianity, Buddhism, Jainism, replace offerings
of the heart, renunciations of the inner self for
the oblations of the ancient; but they ought not
to be replaced but to be added on to the offerings;

all life wherever it is taken strenuously calls for sacrifice, and the ascetic practises of most religions are *Brahma Yajna*, religious exercises that are sacrifices. The Karma Yogi has to continue to strip away whatever accretions to himself he has been tempted to make in daily life by set practices of mortification, the term being used in the western sense of stripping away vain employments, curiosity, fantasies and the like. Towards *Brahma-Yajna* comes in as help the Scripture or representation of the great Law; it does not matter what the Scripture is, provided it is read in the spirit **known** to the Karma Yogi.

LESSON IX

We have provided only for the Karma Yogi who is a man of the world and householder (*Grihasta*), but have not taken note of the Karma Yogi to whom the whole world is a home, who has no other country but the world to which he has devoted himself, to which he has decided to be a servant; what in ancient Hindu parlance is called (the life of a) *Vanaprastha* or recluse. This greater Karma Yogi recognises that the thousands of points of the confused, egotistical, proprietary, partisan, nationalist, life-wasting chaos of human life has to be changed into a coherent development of a kingdom that shall be a kingdom of God. The Karma Yogi has already learned that there can be no such thing as separate existence in the universe; he has understood that all existence is actually one and that one is not the fraction that he once called the "I"; the Karma Yogi has found a way of escape for that fraction of consciousness; he has known that fraction and other such fractions are illusions or delusions, but yet he understands that his own task is unaccomplished while there remains *any* fragment of consciousness thus unemancipated from illusion.

The modern world has progressed far; the optimism and refinement of the modern imagination has changed the attitude of thinkers towards ascetic practices and mortification so that people have begun again to ask as in the days of the *Bhagavad Gita*-religion, what need there is of torment of the violation of the outer nature if the inner dispositions are all right. The Karma Yogi who has mastered the lessons of the *Bhagavad Gita* and of Karma Yoga will look on pleasures and pains, abundance and privation as alike irrelevant and indifferent. He can engage in actions and experience joy without compunction of fear or enslavement or degradation. Our ultra optimistic attitude of today is that we may treat evil by the method of ignoring; man has only to close his eyes to the existence of pain and suffering in the universe outside of himself and he will be quit of it altogether and can sail through life happily on a healthy minded, bias-less basis. But this is a shallow dodge, a mean evasion; pain and wrong and death must be fairly met and overcome in higher excitement or else their sting remains essentially unbroken. If one has ever taken the fact of the prevalence of death into his comprehension —drowning, torture, entombment alive, wild beasts, worse men and hideous diseases—he can with difficulty, it seems to us, continue his own career of worldly prosperity without suspecting that he may, all the while, not be really inside the game. This is what the Karma Yogi thinks and he voluntarily takes the great step—of the *Vani*, wanderer.

In heroism life's supreme mystery is hidden; we tolerate in the modern world no one who has no capacity for it whatever in any direction. On the other hand, whatever a man's frailties may otherwise be, if he be willing to risk death and still more if he risk it heroically in the service he has chosen, that fact consecrates him for ever; if he is able to fling away like a flower his life, caring nothing for it, we account him in the deepest way our born superior; the metaphysical mystery thus recognised by common sense that: he who attacks death that is the eater up of men meets best the secret of the universe, is the secret mystery of asceticism; the folly of the cross so inexplicable by the intellect has yet its indestructible vital meaning.

The world in which this law of vicarious suffering prevails is a far richer and nobler world than one wherein everyone would get his dessert of good or ill; such a world would not be a world in which there could be no sacrifice for another, no little children, no mother love, a world of independent adult individuals each standing up for himself or herself, a moral world without shade or dew where all life was legal because life could not bear another's burdens or hazard all things for another's sake. There can be no difficulty whatever in bringing home to intelligent men that vicarious suffering, the *Purusha Medha* of the *Vedas*, is a law of the nth dimension, a law beyond all laws, beyond time. We are all bearing the suffering of many past centuries and laying down our life for centuries yet to be, for are we not a composite of milliards of lives, lives that some of them have been from of old, others that yet are to be born, for whose sake we really live and die and are born? If we did not incarnate, and if we did not care to be born again and again, what of all these lesser beings, *Bhootas*, that are of us, that would not have been, but for us, that would not have been brought into being or much less have obtained experience?

The practical course of action for us as religious men, as Karma Yogis, would therefore not be to turn our backs on the ascetic impulse, but rather to discover some outlet for it of which the fruits in the way of privation and hardship might be objectively useful. The Karma Yogi has to cease from following his own path to perfection, and yet to find saner channels for the heroism that has been his inspiration. In the West, as regards the laity, athletics, militarism and individual and national enterprise and adventure have been pointed out as the *via media*. War and adventure assuredly keep all who engage in them from treating themselves too tenderly. Discomfort and annoyance, hunger and wet, pain and cold, squalor and filth cease to have any deterrent action whatever; death turns into a commonplace matter and its usual power to check our action vanishes. But in the East, these things have never been and neither hunger nor wet, discomfort nor annoyance daunt the ordinary householder; both for the East and West what is now wanted, say many, is the discovery in the social realm of the moral equivalent of war—something heroic that will speak to one universally as war does and yet will be as compatible with their spiritual selves as war has proved itself incompatible.

What then must be the life work of the Karma Yogi? It must be first of all the Preaching of the Good Law, it must be the dissemination of the Yogi Philosophy and its teachings that have made him a Karma Yogi. His second duty and joy must be to find out in all the great religions the great and good Law, to follow it out in details and to disseminate that knowledge to solace eager souls waiting for it. His third joy must be to preach the kingdom of God as he found it and as he found it not for himself but for all; his fourth joy should be in the reformation of the wandering beggar that is, alas, a disgrace to asceticism; to educate him, to regulate him, to use him wherever found in the world and bring him into the fold firstly of a great religion, if nothing better can be done and then teach him the good Law of "Do what thou wilt." A fifth joy for the Karma Yogi would be to render aid in the regulation of food supply to the masses, the work that the homes for the poor, the Salvation Army shelters, etc., are doing. A sixth, but this can be undertaken only by qualified men, would be medical relief to the poor; though what the Karma Yogi can do is to make medicos help the poor; and ways and means by the many, for salvaging civilisation, can be found in world experience that require no catalogue here.

Of course herein it is taken that the Karma Yogi in this stage has got beyond a home; he has not become yet God; to do that he must have become one who has not the wherewithal to find a place where he may lay down his weary head (*Aniketah* is the term for this stage of Karma Yogi in the *Bhagavad Gita*). The Karma Yogi finds the greater world his home, and all life his brethren; he is a Forester of that great forest the world, *Loka aranya*. All the suggestions made for the forester's life, the *Vanaprastha's asrama* now cruelly forgotten or neglected, may be considered by the Karma Yogi; he may for instance be a householder in the forest but yet have nothing to do with legal positions, or he may have given up the service of fire and have gone forth naked, *nagna*, i.e. without the need of protection against

chills or heat, out into the cold; recognising not
at all the civil law, refusing all the rights that confused modern civilisation still allows to man, the
Karma Yogi can, of course, devote himself to
social service and remain a hermit in the world,
but here he differs from the modern social service
worker in the fact that he has deliberately turned
his back on a house and home and that he combines
social service with true religion, its study and
teaching. The point is that the Karma Yogi continues to work ever more energetically just because he has attained, and makes his work thorough
and exhaustive.

The model that the Karma Yogi, who has become a social worker, keeps before him is that
of our father, the Sun. Before sunrise the Karma
Yogi must have bathed and finished his ablutions
and be ready to adore the Visible God, the Sun.
And for the Adoration, any Rhythm, any simple
prayer would suffice; in Hinduism the Sun in the
early morn *Sandhya* (twilight) prayers is called
Mitra, Friend. God is the Friend; all that the
Karma Yogi meets are Friends, Companions in
the great enterprise called Life, illuminated, nay,
even led, by the Sun that shineth on all alike. All
may draw their warmth from him; to none is he
partial; for he is the Friend. The Karma Yogi,
too, may get the best out of humanity by seeking
its friendliness, by the cheery word, by the kind

thought, by solicitous care, by ignoring unkindness shown in return for kindness. The Karma Yogin can work out for himself how best he may utilise the *Mitra* aspect, the friendliness as a concrete practice, with or without its adjuncts of compassion, benevolence, charity and the like. The various ways in which God the friend was portrayed and adored are to be found in the *Mithra* cults of ancient Persia, to the literature on which we would refer our readers; so much of space would be taken up did we deal with any of the beauties of the teaching.

The sun is both food and raiment to the Karma Yogi in this stage; he may not take any cooked food at all; a fruit and nut diet must be his, for this course of life has to make him independent of all the artificialities of civilisation; he may exist on alms whatever is given him unasked, but he shall not keep by anything for the morrow, for that would make him dependent and fearful. Above all must the Karma Yogi be independent and fearless, regretless, in a sense unrepentant, for he does not need to waste any more thought on the past that he need not recall by vain repentance, and all artificiality, whether of fashion, convention or compunction, has to cease in the natural life of the Karma Yogi who renounces all other clubs than that of the Bohemians or Wanderers.

Just before the mid-day must the Karma Yogi

again bathe and adore our father the Sun again, in some simple prayer as hereunder, a translation of a *Rg* verse rendered into modern language:

> Isvara, Lord of Light! Make us all channels through which thou Pourest! Teach Us to know thine voice and effulgence in other hearts as in ours and inform us with thine radiance time without end, in eternal cycles!

And again must the Karma Yogin just before sunset bathe and adore the Sun, who is *Varuna* this time, *Varuna* the quaintness of the *Rg Veda*, *Varuna* the translated *Ahura Mazda*, *Varuna* the great coil (*pasa*), *Varuna* the harbinger of Night, the Night of rest, the night of dawn, the night when beauty shall retire to reappear in another divine garment of day, *Varuna* the ocean of joy, the refuge that is of the Mother, the sleep divine that cheers but does not kill.

The Karma Yogin has to bathe, to wash himself thoroughly, because he has been living the strenuous life all along every day, throughout the day; he must shed all that, always turning afresh to the beauty of nature dancing before him; the experiences in the violet, orange and ultra violet of the early morn are not the experiences of the "*green*" of mid-day; they are quite different from the red and red-violet of the evening, and each of the experiences has to be met by a fresh appreciation, a fresh dress of the mind, a cleanliness of the embodiment that has to be free from prejudice. And adoring the Sun shall the Karma Yogi offer his service in to the radiance of Truth, *Satyai Jyotishi* to which the sun has transferred on sunset his radiance. The radiance that had been was that of the Oversoul in man our Father the Sun. When he was hid where then had gone the radiance? Why, it was there still, but we can now see it as Truth what was the Sun's glory.

So utterly is the Sun's model to be followed that during the rainy season the Karma Yogi, if a *Vanaprasta* (monastic), was not to travel about at all; he was to stay for the four months minding the insect life that springs luxuriantly in the tropic during the rains, in one place, giving no worry whatever to householders whose bounden duty was long considered to be attention to guests, in India. Of course, all activity periods must be followed by rest periods, as Lent follows ordinary life periods; as the *Ramzan* period breaks the animal life of men. In modern life, therefore, the Karma Yogi may well devote some months of his year to recoupment, study and preparation for fresh activity. But always is the Sun to be his model; every recoupment, every night of the soul must make its conscious activity better and clearer and turn on newer ideals and newer uses to be taken out of life for the sake of the people. "All for the people," shall ever be his motto, as has been repeatedly said.

LESSON X

The type of the Karma Yogi is the sage Janaka who is the topic of many anecdotes. Janaka was a great Emperor and a sage as well, he was the greatest of the Karma Yogis. His empire was called *Mithila;* he was said to be the father of *Queen Seeta,* the wife of *Sri Rama,* one of the incarnations of God in Hindu legend. His empire was also called *Videha.* You can find him referred to in the Buddhist writings and also in Jain works, but in these later as King *Nimi.* It is said of the king that seeing one day his capital city in flames, he said that nothing of him had been destroyed, he still remained of unbounded wealth. "Happy are we, happy live we who call nothing our own; when Mithila is burnt nothing is burnt which belongs to me," says the *Pravargya of King Nimi,* I-9-23, *Uttaradhyayana Sutra* (Jain)—Sacred Book of the East—Max Muller's edition. Similarly says the Dharmpada: "We live happily indeed thought we call nothing our own. We shall be as the bright gods feeding on happiness." Janaka was like the stone that is not flung off the ever whirling wheel of life, *Arishta.* Nemi is his other name in the *Vedic* literature. He was the *chakravarti,* he let things work out their course, he let the wheel (*chakra*) roll on, as had been advised in the *Gita*, III-16.

One of the earliest *Upanishads* explains the rule of life of Janaka in an anecdote: Once upon a time there was a great sage, *Shuka*, a celibate, one born a sage, the son of Vyasa, the sage who rearranged the Hindu scriptures. Though a born sage, much of the world phenomenalising seemed understandable to Shuka and on asking his father was referred to Janaka, King of Mithila. Shuka went to Janaka's palace gate and sent up his name that Vyasa's son Shuka was waiting. Let him wait was the reply, but at the gate Shuka was, however, received with the utmost respect and all hospitality was shown him; for seven days no reply came and Shuka passed into the inner courtyard. There too, though very cordially received, he got no word from Janaka; he then passed into the inner apartments, but could not see the king for another seven days; but girls galore, rich viands and all good things were placed before Shuka for his enjoyment. Shuka was not at all charmed out by any of these; seeing which at the end of seven days Janaka himself came and waited on Shuka. And thereon ensues a conversation in which Janaka explains to Shuka how it is possible to be a Karma Yogi, to accept the universe, to Act and yet not be affected by his actions. Yes, so can you too, Brother aspirant, you too can Act and yet not be affected by your Acts; just as the soldier in obeying his general, the general thinking of the good of the country he serves, while ordering slaughter.

Yes, you can, you ought to, live as the kings and princes crowned and uncrowned of this world have always lived, as masters always live—but let it not be in self indulgence—on the other hand make your self indulgence your religion. The hero, says the *Bhagavad Gita*, plunges into the work of the world, and undertakes his daily duties and pleasures exactly as another but non-hero, un-educated man would; the difference in his case being that he is not moved by his environments or his acts as the other man is. It has always to be recognised that the majority of men in all ages best serve their kind by a life of quiet duty in the family in their daily work, in the support of cer-tain definite philanthropic causes, or in following up great examples—and the Karma Yogi can, of course, choose to belong to and maintain the out-ward conventions of the great majority he is sur-rounded by. The Hindu Yogi philosophy from very ancient days admits of no facile flight to the wilderness, no sterile virtue; indeed it does count the recluse who fasts among scorpions in a cave as no better than a deserter in hiding. Eastern read-ers can read the *Maitrayi Upanishad* (one of the so-called minor *Upanishads*) where it says: "He who after taking the vows abandons his own country is like a thief; selfishness is *the* son, riches are *the* brethren, glamour *the* house, desire *the* wife that one has to give up—thus, giving up these, only, is one freed." It is quite possible, quite permissible, really it *is* advised that the Karma Yogi do remain in the world that he is yet out of. Mind you, you are the master of destiny which is the Harvest of *your* thoughts—not the result of your environments.

There has been here an item of horseplay introduced into the practice of Karma Yoga by many teachers. The Karma Yogin had been told that he must remain behind to help humanity. The Karma Yogin has himself conquered, has become perfectly indifferent, perfectly energetic, perfectly creative; at this stage he gives himself completely up to the service of the universe, not merely of Humanity alone, having become acutely conscious that his own fortunate condition is not shared by that which he now is. It is then, not because of geocentricity, that the Karma Yogi turns his face downwards for he can save himself only by saving others, by preaching the good Law of "Do what thou wilt—*Matha Ischasi Tatha Kuru.*" "Geocentricity," writes M_____, is a very pathetic and amusing childish characteristic of the older schools. There is no reason whatever for imagining that to help humanity is the only kind of work worth doing by the Karma Yogi. Helping humanity is a very nice thing for those who like it and no doubt those who do so deserve well of their fellows. But the feeling of the desire to help humanity is itself a limitation and a drag just as bad as any other—for in the ultimate it is just swinging a censer by ourselves to our supposed moral superiority.

Very true the masses have to pass through a dual transformation; (a) they have to become divorced from every element of exoteric superstition and priestcraft, (b) they have to become educated men enslaved whether by an idea or by other men. But how far the Karma Yogi should interfere so as to bring up humanity to his standard is entirely a matter for himself. There are many dangers in the way; the Karma Yogi must proceed very warily. "The student of occultism must belong to no special creed or sect, yet he is bound to show outward respect to every creed and faith if he would become a Karma Yogi Adept. He must not be bound by the prejudged and sectarian opinions of any one and he has to form his own opinions and come to his own conclusions in accordance with the rules of evidence furnished to him by the science to which he is devoted," says a Teacher. And again, as says Ragon (*Des Initiations*, p. 22): "We have seen in our days 'all through the people, nothing for the people' a false and dangerous system. The real axiom ought to be 'all for the people and with the people; all for the people, nothing through the people'." For the Karma Yogi all that has been advised with regard to helping humanity is that he should adapt every one of his actions, govern each one of his thoughts, frame each one of his words so that it doesn't at all interfere with any one's free will. For every one is a star, a blazing Sun whose destiny none may interfere with.

Of course it is considered an especially sacred duty to instruct all in the doctrines of Yogi Philosophy, especially to teach the Law of "Do what thou wilt," to teach all people independence of character and freedom of thought, and to warn all that servility and cowardice are the most deadly diseases of the soul. "Thou who have not accepted the Law are therefore as it were troglodytes, survivals of a past civilisation to be treated accordingly; kindness should be shown them as to any other animal and every effort made to bring them into freedom," say the Rules. But equally well do some Mystics say: "Be prudent, we say, prudent and wise, and above all take care what those who learn from you believe in: lest by deceiving themselves they deceive others .... for such is the fate of every truth with which men are as yet unfamiliar .... Let rather the super-cosmic and sub-cosmic mysteries remain a dreamland for those who can neither see nor yet believe that others can...."

"Point out the 'way' however dimly, and lost among the host, as does the evening star to those who tread their path in darkness," says the *Voice of the Silence* (Madame H. P. Blavatsky), and again: "Be, O disciple (*Lanoo*) like them (Mercury, Mars and Sun). Give light and comfort to the toiling pilgrims and seek out him who knows still less than thou, who in his wretched desolation sits starving for the bread of wisdom and the bread which feeds the shadow, without a Teacher, Hope or consolation and let him hear the Law."

Most specially is the teaching to be understood as applying to the East where the tyranny of the *Guru Sishya Bhava* has been of telling effect. Knowledge may not be obtained unless from a Teacher, and the Teacher he is as ignorant as he whom he is asked to teach. The world in India is full of the world-gurus, so they style themselves, denying to the poor and down-trodden any rights at all. Everyone has a right to know, and every Karma Yogi has a right to teach, the duty to teach. Every one's first duty is to himself and to his progress in the Path; but his second duty which presses the other hard, is to give assistance to those not so advanced as he.

Indeed, in one place in the Scriptures they say that though the Karma Yogi has found a way for escape (Salvation) for that fraction of consciousness that he called the "I" and though he knows that not only that consciousness but all other consciousness are part of an illusion, yet he feels that his own task is not accomplished while there remains any fragment of consciousness thus unemancipated from illusion. The Karma Yogin having found a Divine Kingdom in himself turns to find out the Divine Purpose in the complex harmony of the External life; for each one *is* free to live as he will and the luxury of this enjoyment is such that he becomes careful to avoid the disturbance of the equal rights of others. Yes, all objects in their activity, substance and form indicate their relationship and thereby their usefulness to all other things and the phenomena of psychical research indicate that there is absolute connection between *Minds* here and now existing in ways over and beyond those accounted for by the senses; though our ordinary normal consciousness are severed from each other and apparently distinct so that though we communicate with each other through speech and writing, we are nevertheless in connection with each other in subliminal levels. It can thus be seen that the Karma Yogi may not encourage, notice or make any difference between any one thing and any other thing. He may not confound the space, marks saying they are one, they are many.

Yes, to each the knowledge of his Infinite Will,
his Destiny to perform the Great Work, the reali-
sation of his true Self; aye, be he barber or cobbler,
or Brahmin or Pariah, to each again will come the
knowledge of his finite will whereby one is
Prophet, one poet, one worker in jade, another
worker in steel. Every one is unfettered to think,
to revel in the Great Act, each one is a God, did
he but know it; each one is saved, did he but
realise it! And as each one binds himself and
takes his pleasure does he remain blacksmith,
cobbler, barber—never when his soul revolts. In
everything so ever inhereth its own perfection
proper to it and to neglect its full operation bring-
eth distortion to the whole. Act therefore in all
ways, Karma Yogi, but transforming the effect
of all these ways to the one way of God. I am
translating verses XVIII, 45 and 46 of the
Bhagavad Gita.

In the commentary on these verses, the found-
ers of the creeds of Modern Hinduism are alike
in one view about *Sva Karma*, one's own Karma.
Of the Karma Yogi, Ramanuja has it that man
attains perfection, i.e. attains God by God's grace
granted when he worships God as the inner soul
abiding in every object of worship, God by whom
all things are pervaded. According to Sankara,
all activity (*Pravritti*) proceeds from Isvara, the
Antaryamin, the Ruler Within. Worshipping the

Lord, says Sankara, by one's Acts (Thoughts), man attains the perfection of the *Jnana Nishta,* the willing "Death." Madhavacharya says that by one's Acts of Worship of the Lord one obtains *Jnana* (Intuitive Appreciation) and next Salvation. *Sva Karma* is with all these the worship of the Lord God, the true function of the real Ego (*Sva*) in man. That is what the Karma Yogi has to bear in mind, namely that all Act is a Sacrament, must be as a sacrament, and as naught else than a sacrament; not merely to hold the view but to turn one's commonest acts into sacraments is the work of the Karma Yogin, to make his very self-indulgence his religion. He may drink but he shall drink to the glory of God; not to make himself besotted. He shall pick up all the flowers by the roadside in humble *Pooja* (worship) at the Throne of God the Invisible King behind the darkness of the Threshold of Life. Indeed, those who, whether they eat or drink or whatever they do, do all to the glory of God, may be said to turn their commonest acts into sacraments. Read carefully verse IX-27 of the *Bhagavad Gita,* any translation, and make it the *Mantra* for this Lesson.

> "Whatever Thine Act, what thou consumest;
> What thou sacrificeth; what thou granteth,
> What thou yearneth after, do it to the glory
> of God."

Let every act of thine be a magical exercise.

LESSON XI

Some lessons back we told you of the factors governing each act, of how the factors were the sphere of the act, the enjoyer of the act (3), the various agents or instruments used in the act (4), the various forms in which the act came to be (*Cheshta*) together with destiny or *daiva,* God the marginal error, the cumulative power of space-time, of the whole universe as a fifth. We told you specially that consequently it would be foolish to assume that any one by himself could be the Actor; we again said that none the less the Individual was possessed of the fullest freewill and that he ought to do only as he wilt. How the position we took up was in no sense self-contradictory we have mentioned in prior chapters but here we shall further state the great need, the very great need, there is for the exhibition of one's Freewill every moment of one's life. Albeit destiny be all potent as being the will of Many, it is none the less to be understood by the Karma Yogi that he too is a many in one that his will too is the will of many of him; when both wills become identical the result is sudden and favorable.

But if on the contrary the will of the individual had been unconsciously against the will of the universe, what happens? Is Thought a waste? Are not motives of any account in this divine harmony that we call the universe? Can it be that man thinking good thoughts all along, but defeated at every moment by circumstances, is to find his life a waste? No, says the Hindu-Yogi Philosophy. The subconscious incubation of the motives deposited by the experience of life when ripe do burst into flower, says the *Bhagavad Gita*, the text book *par excellence* of Karma Yogi. Thoughts are never waste; you can pile on your good intentions and good thoughts till the cumulative effect, as in all *mantras*, affirmations, magick, becomes of powerful effect breaking down all obstacles before the fruition of the good thought. The last straw breaks the camel's back, says the proverb; if in alchemy you add one more atom-ion to make up of the valency of the element, it breaks up and disintegrates as seen in radio metallurgy. Read what Madame H. P. Blavatsky says in the *Voice of the Silence*, part 3, the seven portals.

"70. Remember tho that fightest for man's liberation each failure is success and each sincere attempt wins its reward in time. The holy germs that sprout and grow unseen in the disciple's soul their stalks wax strong at each new trial, they bend like reeds but never break nor can they ever be lost .... But when the hour has struck they blossom forth."

Yes, it is very difficult to continue practising

Karma Yogi of all the Yogas because very often very little advancement is seen apparently for a very long time. To quote a familiar instance,— there is water on the fire and nothing whatever happens or appears to be happening; but one continues to keep it on the fire, and lo! without warning it suddenly boils. You may get the temperature to 99 degrees and keep it at 99 degrees for a thousand years and the water will not boil. It is the last step that does the trick. Similarly in the practices given herein it may be said that one must be prepared to accept that the *mantra* or practice one has been doing, however bad, is the best one can go on with, and no attempt to change *mantra* after *mantra* can be encouraged by us. Such students are given up by us as perfectly hopeless.

There is an aspect of the doctrine of Detachment that has been rediscovered in the West and may be found, as "art for art's sake." Actually it is an indifference especially necessary when wrong thoughts come and afflict one and attempt to persuade one that if one goes on the Path of Karma Yoga he will go mad or some such thing. Says Frater O. M.: "In times of dryness the 'Devil' comes to you and persuades you that it is most necessary for your spiritual progress to repose (i.e. refrain from the task of the Karma Yogi). He will explain that by the great law of action and reaction you should alternate the task you have set forth to do with something else, that you should in fact somehow or other change your plans. Any attempt to argue with him will assuredly result in defeat. You must be able to reply: "But I am not in the least interested in my further progress; I am doing this because I have set it down in my programme to do it. It may hurt my spiritual progress more than anything in the world. That does not matter. I will be gladly damned eternally but I will not break my obligation in the smallest detail. By doing thus you come out at the other end and discover that the whole controversy was illusion."

This is the experience of the ordinary Yogi; the Karma Yogi's position is harder. As Steiner says in his "Initiation" the Karma Yogi "finds no definite goal to be reached; all is left in his own hands; he finds himself in a situation where nothing occasions him to act. He must find his way all alone and from out of himself. And he must be able to attain always the point of being able when confronted suddenly with some task or problem demanding immediate attention to come to a swift conclusion, to act without delay or personal consideration or any the least hesitation. Nothing or nobody need give him the strength he needs but himself alone."

As says H. G. Wells: "It is the amazing and

distressful discovery of every believer that one can find himself caught unawares by a base impulse; he then discovers that discontinuousness of our apparently homogeneous selves, the unincorporated and warring elements that seemed altogether absent; we are tripped up by forgetfulness, by distraction, by old habits, by tricks of appearance; there come dull patches of existence; those mysterious obliterations of one's finer sense that are due at times to the little minor poisons that one eats or drinks, to phases of fatigue, ill health or bodily disorder or one is betrayed by some unanticipated storm of emotion brewed deep in the animal being and released by any trifling discontent such as personal jealousy or one is relaxed by contentment into vanity."

We may call the group of ideas to which man devotes himself and from which he works the "habitual center of his personal energy. It makes a great difference to a man whether one set of ideas or another be the center of his energy; and it makes a great difference as regards any set of ideas which he may possess whether they become central or remain peripheral in him," says James, the pragmatic; but even this definition would not apply to the Karma Yogi who has always to have a changing center, who has to change the center of his point of view and cultivate his appreciation sufficiently widely so as to cover the innumerable

experiences of the world; for in every sense the
Karma Yogi is truly homeless and these regula-
tions and observations that apply in an ego-centric
metaphysic do not apply to him at all.   And this
change of center of point of view *is* his Karma
Yoga.

Mistakes do not afflict the Karma Yogi in the
least; no, not even the fact that he has in the immediate to go against the Law of Karma; he does
not care, he breaks the law and suffers the reaction, but he has done what he had obligated himself to do.   The Karma Yogi of all yogis is not
ever in training; rules and prohibitions for other
stages of Yoga for the *mantra* yogi, *raja* yogi,
sparsa yogi, *abhava* yogi, etc., have no meaning in
his case.   In these cases the would-be yogins are
in training; and in their case prohibitions are made
general rules; but the rules do not apply to people
not under training, never to people beyond the
need for further *yogaic* training.   To break training is not a sin for any one who is not in training;
the Karma Yogi is a ceaseless worker who is not
only not less than a man but *more* than one.

The Karma Yogi in such a complexity has always to be watchful (*atmavan*).   The watchfulness is to be very active, a watchfulness at the door
of one's thought, never off guard, but all the while
there is being cultivated an inner indifference, a
faith that mountains cannot shake.   Apparently

the Karma Yogi is silent, for he is able to inhibit thought; actually thought from the universe surges through him, strengthens him and perhaps leaves its traces behind in rendering him every moment more useful in sensing.

PEACE UNTO ALL BEINGS

The Complete Works

of

YOGI RAMACHARAKA

SCIENCE OF BREATH

FOURTEEN LESSONS—YOGI PHILOSOPHY

ADVANCED COURSE IN YOGI PHILOSOPHY

RAJA YOGA

GNANI YOGA

PHILOSOPHIES AND RELIGIONS OF INDIA

HATHA YOGA

PSYCHIC HEALING

MYSTIC CHRISTIANITY

LIFE BEYOND DEATH

BHAGAVAD GITA

THE SPIRIT OF THE UPANISHADS

PRACTICAL WATER CURE